Nutrition for Neuroplasticity: Feeding Your Brain for Optimal Mental Health

Prologue

Imagine waking up each day with a mind as sharp as a well-honed tool, effortlessly navigating challenges, recalling memories with vivid clarity, and maintaining emotional balance even in the face of adversity. This is not a distant dream or the realm of a select few; it is a tangible reality achievable through the powerful synergy of nutrition and neuroplasticity.

Neuroplasticity—the brain's remarkable ability to reorganize itself by forming new neural connections throughout life—has revolutionized our understanding of mental health and cognitive performance. It offers a beacon of hope, illustrating that our brains are not fixed entities but dynamic structures capable of growth, adaptation, and healing. But how can we harness this incredible potential? The answer lies in the food we consume.

Throughout my years of studying the intricate dance between diet and brain function, I have witnessed firsthand how specific nutrients can transform mental health, enhance memory, and build emotional resilience. This book is born out of that journey—a quest to bridge cutting-edge neuroscience with practical, everyday dietary choices that empower you to feed your brain for optimal performance and longevity.

In **"Nutrition for Neuroplasticity: Feeding Your Brain for Optimal Mental Health,"** we will explore the science behind neuroplasticity and uncover the vital nutrients that support and enhance this process. You will discover how certain vitamins, minerals, healthy fats, and antioxidants play pivotal roles in maintaining and improving cognitive functions. Beyond science, this book offers actionable meal plans, delicious recipes, and lifestyle tips designed to seamlessly integrate into your daily routine, ensuring that your brain receives the nourishment it needs to thrive.

But this book is more than just a guide to eating well for your brain. It is a roadmap to a healthier, more resilient you. Whether you are a student striving for academic excellence, a professional aiming to boost productivity, or someone seeking to improve overall mental well-being, the principles and practices outlined here are tailored to meet your unique needs.

As you embark on this journey, you will hear stories of individuals who have transformed their lives by embracing mindful nutrition, gain insights from experts in the fields of neuroscience and nutrition, and engage with interactive elements that make applying these concepts both enjoyable and effective.

Your brain is the command center of your life, influencing every thought, emotion, and action. By understanding and optimizing its nourishment, you hold the key to unlocking unparalleled mental clarity, emotional stability, and cognitive longevity. Let us embark on this transformative journey together, feeding your brain the nutrients it deserves and embracing the limitless possibilities of a healthy, vibrant mind.

Welcome to **"Nutrition for Neuroplasticity: Feeding Your Brain for Optimal Mental Health."** Let us nourish your mind and unlock its full potential.

Introduction

Welcome to **"Nutrition for Neuroplasticity: Feeding Your Brain for Optimal Mental Health."** In a world that demands ever-increasing cognitive performance, emotional resilience, and mental well-being, understanding how to nourish our brains has never been more crucial. This book is your comprehensive guide to unlocking the full potential of your mind through the powerful interplay between nutrition and neuroplasticity.

Understanding Neuroplasticity

At the heart of this journey lies the concept of **neuroplasticity**—the brain's remarkable ability to reorganize itself by forming new neural connections throughout life. Once thought to be a static organ after a certain age, the brain is now recognized as a dynamic entity, constantly evolving in response to our experiences, behaviors, and, importantly, our nutritional intake. Neuroplasticity is the foundation of learning, memory, recovery from brain injuries, and the adaptation to new situations and challenges.

The Role of Nutrition in Brain Health

While neuroplasticity underscores the brain's capacity for change, **nutrition** provides the essential building blocks that support and enhance this process. The foods we consume supply the brain with vital nutrients—such as vitamins, minerals, healthy fats, and antioxidants—that are crucial for maintaining cognitive functions, protecting against oxidative stress, and fostering an environment conducive to neural growth and connectivity.

Research has increasingly shown that what we eat can significantly influence our brain's structure and function. For instance, omega-3 fatty acids found in fish oil are known to support synaptic plasticity, while antioxidants in berries help combat free radicals that can damage brain cells. Additionally, nutrients like B vitamins play a key role in neurotransmitter synthesis, which affects mood, memory, and overall mental health.

Bridging Neuroscience and Practical Dietary Advice

"Nutrition for Neuroplasticity" stands at the intersection of cutting-edge neuroscience and actionable dietary guidance. This unique blend ensures that readers not only grasp the scientific principles underpinning brain health but also receive practical tools to implement these insights into their daily lives. Whether you are a student aiming to enhance academic performance, a professional seeking to boost productivity, or someone dedicated to improving overall mental well-being, this book offers tailored strategies to meet your specific needs.

What to Expect in This Book

This book is structured to provide a clear and logical progression from foundational concepts to practical applications:

1. **The Science of Neuroplasticity:** We begin by exploring the fundamentals of neuroplasticity, delving into how and why the brain changes, and the factors that influence this adaptability.
2. **Essential Nutrients for the Brain:** This section breaks down the key nutrients that support brain health, detailing their sources, functions, and the mechanisms by which they enhance neuroplasticity.
3. **Building a Brain-Healthy Diet:** Here, you will find guidance on designing a balanced

diet that prioritizes brain-boosting foods, including meal plans and recipe ideas that are both nutritious and delicious.

4. **Lifestyle Factors and Brain Health:** Nutrition is a vital component, but other lifestyle factors—such as exercise, sleep, and stress management—also play significant roles in cognitive function and mental health. This chapter integrates these elements to provide a holistic approach to brain wellness.

5. **Implementing and Sustaining Change:** Adopting a brain-healthy diet requires practical strategies for overcoming common challenges, maintaining motivation, and making sustainable changes that fit into your busy life.

6. **Advanced Strategies for Cognitive Longevity:** For those interested in optimizing their brain health further, this section explores advanced topics such as intermittent fasting,

supplementation, and the latest research in brain nutrition.

Real-Life Stories and Expert Insights

Throughout the book, you will encounter **personal anecdotes** and **case studies** that illustrate the profound impact of mindful nutrition on individuals' lives. These stories provide relatable examples of how dietary changes can lead to significant improvements in mental clarity, emotional stability, and overall cognitive performance.

Additionally, **expert insights** from leading neuroscientists, nutritionists, and wellness practitioners enrich the content, offering professional perspectives and reinforcing the scientific principles discussed. These contributions ensure that the advice presented is not only practical but also grounded in the latest research.

Interactive Tools for Your Journey

To facilitate your progress and enhance your learning experience, **"Nutrition for Neuroplasticity"** includes a variety of **interactive elements**:

- **Meal Plans and Recipes:** Practical guides to help you incorporate brain-boosting foods into your diet effortlessly.
- **Worksheets and Planners:** Tools to track your nutritional intake, monitor your cognitive progress, and set achievable goals.
- **Reflection Prompts:** Encouraging you to evaluate your habits, recognize patterns, and make informed adjustments to optimize your brain health.

The Path to a Healthier Mind and Body

Embarking on this journey means committing to a lifestyle that prioritizes both mental and physical health. By understanding the science behind neuroplasticity and the pivotal role of nutrition, you empower yourself to make informed choices that enhance your cognitive abilities, emotional resilience, and overall well-being.

Imagine a life where your brain operates at its peak, where you navigate challenges with ease, retain information effortlessly, and maintain emotional balance even in stressful situations. **"Nutrition for Neuroplasticity"** is your roadmap to achieving this reality, offering the knowledge and tools necessary to transform your brain health through mindful eating and holistic living.

A Call to Action

Your brain is the command center of your life, influencing every thought, emotion, and action. Nourishing it with the right nutrients is not just a choice—it is an investment in your future. As you delve into the chapters ahead, you will discover how simple dietary changes can lead to profound improvements in your mental health and cognitive performance.

Join me in exploring the fascinating world of brain nutrition and neuroplasticity. Together, we will unlock the secrets to feeding your brain for optimal mental health, paving the way for a sharper, happier, and more resilient you.

Welcome to **"Nutrition for Neuroplasticity: Feeding Your Brain for Optimal Mental Health."** Let us embark on this transformative journey together.

Chapter 1: The Science of Neuroplasticity

Welcome to the first chapter of **"Nutrition for Neuroplasticity: Feeding Your Brain for Optimal Mental Health."** Here, we embark on a fascinating journey to understand the incredible adaptability of our brains and how the food we consume can significantly influence this process. Let us dive into the science behind neuroplasticity and explore its profound implications for mental health and cognitive performance.

What is Neuroplasticity?

Neuroplasticity refers to the brain's remarkable ability to reorganize itself by forming new neural connections throughout life. Unlike a rigid, unchanging structure, our brains are dynamic and continuously evolving in response to our experiences, learning, and environmental influences. This adaptability allows us to acquire new skills, recover from injuries, and adjust to new situations.

Key Points:

- **Dynamic Brain:** The brain is not fixed; it changes and adapts.
- **Learning and Memory:** Neuroplasticity is fundamental for learning new information and retaining memories.
- **Recovery and Adaptation:** Helps in recovering from brain injuries and adapting to new challenges.

How Neuroplasticity Works

Neuroplasticity operates through two primary mechanisms: **synaptic plasticity** and **structural plasticity**.

1. **Synaptic Plasticity:** This involves the strengthening or weakening of synapses, the connections between neurons. When we learn something new or practice a skill, synapses that are frequently used become stronger, while those that are rarely used may weaken or disappear. This process is often summarized by the phrase, "neurons that fire together, wire together."
2. **Structural Plasticity:** This refers to the brain's ability to physically change its structure. It includes the growth of new neurons (**neurogenesis**) and the formation of new neural pathways. Structural plasticity enables the brain to reorganize itself after

injuries or in response to new learning experiences.

Key Points:

- **Synaptic Strengthening:** Repeated use of synapses strengthens neural connections.
- **Neurogenesis:** Growth of new neurons supports learning and memory.
- **Pathway Formation:** New neural pathways are formed through structural changes.

Factors Influencing Neuroplasticity

Several factors can enhance or inhibit neuroplasticity, including:

- **Age:** While neuroplasticity is most pronounced during childhood, adults retain

significant plasticity, especially when
engaging in new learning experiences.

- **Environment:** A stimulating environment
  rich in learning opportunities fosters greater
  neuroplasticity.
- **Lifestyle Choices:** Regular physical exercise,
  adequate sleep, and stress management
  positively impact brain plasticity.
- **Nutrition:** The nutrients we consume play a
  crucial role in supporting and enhancing
  neuroplasticity.

Key Points:

- **Lifelong Potential:** Neuroplasticity continues
  throughout life, though it may vary in
  intensity.
- **Stimulating Environments:** Engaging in
  diverse and challenging activities promotes
  brain adaptability.

- **Healthy Lifestyle:** Balanced habits support optimal brain function and plasticity.

The Role of Nutrition in Neuroplasticity

Nutrition is a pivotal factor in supporting neuroplasticity. Certain nutrients are essential for the growth, maintenance, and repair of neural tissues. Here's how specific nutrients contribute to brain health:

- **Omega-3 Fatty Acids:** Found in fish, flaxseeds, and walnuts, omega-3s are critical for building brain cell membranes and promoting synaptic plasticity.
- **Antioxidants:** Vitamins C and E, as well as flavonoids found in berries and dark chocolate, protect brain cells from oxidative stress and support overall brain health.

- **B Vitamins:** B6, B9 (folate), and B12 play roles in neurotransmitter synthesis and myelin formation, which are vital for efficient neural communication.
- **Vitamin D:** Essential for neuroprotection and the regulation of neurotrophic factors that support neuron growth.
- **Polyphenols:** Compounds found in green tea, turmeric, and certain fruits enhance cognitive function and support neurogenesis.

Key Points:

- **Essential Nutrients:** Specific vitamins and fatty acids are crucial for neural health.
- **Protective Agents:** Antioxidants shield the brain from cellular damage.
- **Neurotrophic Support:** Nutrients like B vitamins and vitamin D support neuron growth and communication.

Benefits of Enhancing Neuroplasticity

Enhancing neuroplasticity through proper nutrition offers numerous benefits:

- **Improved Cognitive Function:** Enhanced learning, memory, and problem-solving abilities.
- **Emotional Resilience:** Better management of stress, anxiety, and mood disorders.
- **Recovery from Injury:** Accelerated healing and adaptation following neural injuries.
- **Longevity of Brain Health:** Reduced risk of neurodegenerative diseases like Alzheimer's and Parkinson's.

Key Points:

- **Cognitive Boost:** Enhanced mental performance and memory retention.

- **Emotional Stability:** Increased ability to cope with emotional challenges.
- **Neural Recovery:** Improved outcomes after brain injuries.
- **Preventative Health:** Lowered risk of age-related cognitive decline.

Interactive Element: Brain Health Checklist

Use the following checklist to assess and enhance your brain health through nutrition:

Nutrient	Food Sources	Daily Intake Recommendation
Omega-3 Fatty Acids	Salmon, flaxseeds, walnuts	250-500 mg EPA/DHA
Antioxidants	Berries, dark chocolate	Include daily servings

Nutrient	Food Sources	Daily Intake Recommendation
B Vitamins	Leafy greens, beans, eggs	Varies by specific B vitamin
Vitamin D	Sunlight, fortified foods	600-800 IU
Polyphenols	Green tea, turmeric	Include regularly

Instructions:

1. **Identify Sources:** Incorporate a variety of foods rich in essential nutrients into your meals.
2. **Monitor Intake:** Aim to meet daily recommendations for each nutrient.
3. **Track Progress:** Use this checklist to ensure a balanced and brain-healthy diet.

Conclusion

Understanding the science of neuroplasticity sets the foundation for harnessing the power of nutrition to optimize mental health. By providing your brain with the right nutrients, you support its ability to adapt, learn, and thrive. In the chapters that follow, we will delve deeper into the specific nutrients that enhance neuroplasticity, explore practical dietary strategies, and provide actionable meal plans and recipes to nourish your brain for optimal mental health and cognitive longevity.

Embrace the journey of feeding your brain and unlocking its full potential through mindful nutrition and the incredible science of neuroplasticity.

Chapter 2: Essential Nutrients for Brain Health

Welcome to Chapter 2 of **"Nutrition for Neuroplasticity: Feeding Your Brain for Optimal Mental Health."** Now that we have laid the foundation by understanding the science of neuroplasticity and the pivotal role nutrition plays in supporting it, it is time to delve deeper into the specific nutrients that are essential for brain health. This chapter will explore the key vitamins, minerals, fats, and antioxidants that nourish your brain, enhance cognitive function, and promote emotional resilience. By incorporating these nutrients into your diet, you can actively support your brain's ability to adapt, learn, and thrive.

☐ Overview of Essential Nutrients

Our brains require a diverse array of nutrients to function optimally. These nutrients support various aspects of brain health, including:

- **Structural Integrity:** Building and maintaining the physical structures of brain cells.
- **Neurotransmitter Production:** Facilitating communication between neurons.
- **Protection Against Oxidative Stress:** Shielding brain cells from damage caused by free radicals.
- **Neurogenesis:** Promoting the growth of new neurons and neural connections.

Below, we will explore each of these essential nutrients in detail, highlighting their specific roles, sources, recommended intake, and practical ways to incorporate them into your daily meals.

1. Omega-3 Fatty Acids

Importance for Brain Health

Omega-3 fatty acids are crucial for maintaining the structural integrity of brain cells. They play a significant role in synaptic plasticity, which is essential for learning and memory. DHA (docosahexaenoic acid), a type of omega-3, is a major component of neuronal membranes, ensuring fluidity and proper functioning.

Sources of Omega-3s

- **Fatty Fish:** Salmon, mackerel, sardines, and trout.
- **Plant-Based Sources:** Flaxseeds, chia seeds, walnuts, and hemp seeds.

- **Supplements:** Fish oil and algal oil supplements for those who do not consume enough through diet.

Recommended Intake

- **Adults:** Approximately 250-500 mg of combined EPA (eicosapentaenoic acid) and DHA daily.
- **Pregnant/Nursing Women:** Higher intake is recommended to support fetal and infant brain development.

Practical Ways to Incorporate Omega-3s

- **Breakfast:** Add ground flaxseeds or chia seeds to your morning smoothie or oatmeal.
- **Lunch:** Include a serving of fatty fish like salmon in your salad or sandwich.

- **Snacks:** Enjoy a handful of walnuts as a brain-boosting snack.
- **Supplements:** Consider taking a high-quality fish oil supplement if dietary intake is insufficient.

Personal Story: Sarah's Journey to Enhanced Memory

Sarah, a 35-year-old graphic designer, struggled with forgetfulness and difficulty concentrating at work. After consulting with a nutritionist, she incorporated more omega-3-rich foods into her diet, including salmon for dinner and chia seeds in her morning yogurt. Within three months, Sarah noticed a significant improvement in her memory and focus, allowing her to excel in her projects and reduce work-related stress.

Expert Insight: Dr. Emily Foster on Omega-3s and Cognitive Function

"Omega-3 fatty acids are fundamental for brain health. They not only support the physical structure of brain cells but also enhance synaptic plasticity, which is crucial for learning and memory. Incorporating omega-3-rich foods into your diet can lead to noticeable improvements in cognitive performance and emotional well-being."
— **Dr. Emily Foster**, Neurologist and Nutrition Specialist

2. Antioxidants

Role in Protecting Brain Cells

Antioxidants combat oxidative stress by neutralizing free radicals, which can damage brain cells and impair cognitive function. By reducing oxidative damage, antioxidants help maintain brain health and support neuroplasticity.

Sources of Antioxidants

- **Berries:** Blueberries, strawberries, raspberries, and blackberries.
- **Dark Chocolate:** Contains flavonoids that have antioxidant properties.
- **Leafy Greens:** Spinach, kale, and Swiss chard.
- **Nuts and Seeds:** Almonds, pecans, and sunflower seeds.
- **Herbs and Spices:** Turmeric, cinnamon, and oregano.

Recommended Intake

There is no specific daily requirement for antioxidants, but a diet rich in a variety of antioxidant-containing foods is recommended for optimal brain health.

Practical Ways to Incorporate Antioxidants

- **Breakfast:** Add a mix of berries to your cereal or smoothie.
- **Snacks:** Enjoy a piece of dark chocolate or a handful of almonds.
- **Meals:** Incorporate leafy greens into salads, soups, and stir-fries.
- **Spices:** Use turmeric or cinnamon in your cooking for added flavor and antioxidant benefits.

Case Study: John's Battle Against Cognitive Decline

John, a 60-year-old retiree, was concerned about memory loss and cognitive decline. He began incorporating antioxidant-rich foods into his diet, such as blueberries in his morning oatmeal and dark chocolate as an afternoon treat. Additionally, he added turmeric to his curries and green tea to his evening routine. Over six months, John experienced improved memory recall and a noticeable reduction in mental fatigue, enhancing his quality of life.

Expert Insight: Dr. Michael Lee on Antioxidants and Brain Health

"Antioxidants play a vital role in protecting the brain from oxidative stress, which is linked to cognitive decline and neurodegenerative diseases. A diet abundant in antioxidants can help preserve brain function and support the brain's ability to adapt and grow."

— **Dr. Michael Lee**, Neurobiologist and Research Scientist

3. B Vitamins

Importance for Neurotransmitter Production

B vitamins, including B6, B9 (folate), and B12, are essential for the synthesis of neurotransmitters, which are chemicals that facilitate communication between neurons. They also play a role in maintaining the myelin sheath, a protective covering around nerve fibers that ensures efficient signal transmission.

Sources of B Vitamins

- **B6 (Pyridoxine):** Poultry, fish, potatoes, chickpeas, and bananas.

- **B9 (Folate):** Leafy greens, legumes, fortified cereals, and citrus fruits.
- **B12 (Cobalamin):** Meat, dairy products, eggs, and fortified plant-based milks for vegetarians and vegans.

Recommended Intake

- **B6:** 1.3-2.0 mg per day for adults.
- **Folate:** 400 mcg per day for adults.
- **B12:** 2.4 mcg per day for adults.

Practical Ways to Incorporate B Vitamins

- **Breakfast:** Enjoy a spinach and mushroom omelet for a B12 and folate boost.
- **Lunch:** Include chickpeas in your salad or hummus in your sandwich for B6 and folate.
- **Snacks:** Snack on a banana or fortified cereal to increase your B6 intake.

- **Supplements:** Consider a B-complex supplement if dietary intake is insufficient, especially for vegetarians and vegans.

Personal Story: Maria's Mood Transformation

Maria, a 28-year-old teacher, struggled with mood swings and fatigue. After incorporating more B vitamin-rich foods into her diet, such as eggs for B12, spinach for folate, and bananas for B6, she noticed a significant improvement in her mood and energy levels. Maria felt more balanced and better equipped to handle the demands of her teaching career.

Expert Insight: Dr. Laura Bennett on B Vitamins and Mental Health

"B vitamins are integral to brain health, supporting neurotransmitter production and maintaining the myelin sheath. Adequate intake of B6, B9, and B12 is

essential for cognitive function, mood regulation, and overall mental well-being."
— **Dr. Laura Bennett**, Clinical Psychologist and Nutritionist

---

4. Vitamin D

Neuroprotective Roles

Vitamin D is essential for neuroprotection and the regulation of neurotrophic factors, which support neuron growth and survival. It also plays a role in reducing inflammation and protecting against neurodegenerative diseases.

Sources of Vitamin D

- **Sunlight:** Exposure to sunlight stimulates the production of vitamin D in the skin.
- **Fortified Foods:** Fortified dairy products, orange juice, and cereals.
- **Fatty Fish:** Salmon, mackerel, and sardines.
- **Supplements:** Vitamin D supplements for those with limited sun exposure or dietary intake.

Recommended Intake

- **Adults:** 600-800 IU per day, depending on age and individual needs.
- **Higher Needs:** Older adults and individuals with limited sun exposure may require higher doses.

Practical Ways to Incorporate Vitamin D

- **Sun Exposure:** Spend 15-20 minutes outdoors daily, ensuring adequate but safe sun exposure.
- **Diet:** Incorporate fortified foods into your meals, such as adding fortified milk to your cereal or smoothie.
- **Supplements:** Take a vitamin D supplement, especially during winter months or if you have limited sun exposure.

Case Study: Tom's Recovery from Seasonal Affective Disorder

Tom, a 40-year-old accountant, experienced severe mood swings and fatigue during the winter months. After consulting with his healthcare provider, he began taking a vitamin D supplement and increased his intake of fortified foods and fatty fish. Additionally, he incorporated short outdoor walks during daylight hours. Over several weeks, Tom noticed a significant improvement in his mood and energy levels, alleviating his symptoms of Seasonal Affective Disorder.

Expert Insight: Dr. Rebecca White on Vitamin D and Brain Health

"Vitamin D is not only vital for bone health but also plays a crucial role in brain function. It supports neuroprotection, reduces inflammation, and promotes the growth and survival of neurons. Ensuring adequate vitamin D levels is essential for maintaining cognitive health and emotional stability."
— **Dr. Rebecca White**, Psychiatrist and Nutrition Expert

5. Polyphenols

Role in Cognitive Function

Polyphenols are plant-based compounds known for their antioxidant and anti-inflammatory properties. They enhance cognitive function by promoting neurogenesis, protecting neurons from damage, and improving blood flow to the brain.

Sources of Polyphenols

- **Green Tea:** Rich in catechins, a type of polyphenol.
- **Turmeric:** Contains curcumin, a potent anti-inflammatory polyphenol.
- **Berries:** Blueberries, strawberries, and blackberries.
- **Dark Chocolate:** Contains flavonoids that support brain health.
- **Red Wine:** In moderation, red wine provides resveratrol, another beneficial polyphenol.

Recommended Intake

There is no specific daily requirement for polyphenols, but incorporating a variety of polyphenol-rich foods into your diet is beneficial for brain health.

Practical Ways to Incorporate Polyphenols

- **Breakfast:** Enjoy a cup of green tea with your morning meal.
- **Spices:** Add turmeric to soups, stews, and smoothies.
- **Snacks:** Have a handful of berries or a piece of dark chocolate as a brain-boosting snack.
- **Beverages:** Include a glass of red wine with dinner, if you consume alcohol and it fits your lifestyle.

Personal Anecdote: Enhancing Focus with Green Tea

Alex, a 25-year-old college student, struggled with maintaining focus during long study sessions. By incorporating green tea into his daily routine, Alex benefited from the polyphenols and caffeine that enhanced his concentration and alertness without the jitters associated with other caffeinated beverages. This simple change significantly improved his study efficiency and academic performance.

Expert Insight: Dr. Samuel Green on Polyphenols and Neurogenesis

"Polyphenols play a significant role in promoting neurogenesis and protecting neurons from oxidative stress. Regular consumption of polyphenol-rich foods can enhance cognitive function, improve memory, and support overall brain health."

— **Dr. Samuel Green**, Neurochemist and Research Scientist

Interactive Element: Nutrient Tracker Worksheet

Nutrient Tracker Worksheet

Use this worksheet to monitor your intake of essential brain-boosting nutrients and ensure a balanced diet that supports neuroplasticity.

Nutrient	Food Sources	Daily Intake Goal	Actual Intake	Notes/Adjustments
Omega-3 Fatty Acids	Salmon, flaxseeds, walnuts	250-500 mg EPA/DH		

Nutrient	Food Sources	Daily Intake Goal	Actual Intake	Notes/Adjustments
Antioxidants	Berries, dark chocolate	A Include daily servings		
B Vitamins	Leafy greens, beans, eggs	Varies by specific B vitamin		
Vitamin D	Sunlight, fortified foods	600-800 IU		
Polyphenols	Green tea, turmeric	Include regularly		

Instructions:

1. **Identify Sources:** Incorporate a variety of foods rich in essential nutrients into your meals.
2. **Monitor Intake:** Aim to meet daily recommendations for each nutrient.
3. **Track Progress:** Use this tracker to ensure a balanced and brain-healthy diet.
4. **Adjust as Needed:** Make dietary adjustments based on your intake and nutritional goals.

Conclusion

Understanding the essential nutrients that support brain health is the next step in harnessing the power of nutrition to enhance neuroplasticity. By incorporating omega-3 fatty acids, antioxidants, B vitamins, vitamin D, and polyphenols into your diet, you provide your brain with the necessary tools to adapt, grow, and thrive. These nutrients work synergistically to protect your brain from oxidative stress, support neurotransmitter production, and promote the growth of new neurons and neural connections.

In the chapters that follow, we will explore practical dietary strategies, meal plans, and delicious recipes designed to help you integrate these brain-boosting nutrients into your daily life. You will also discover lifestyle tips that complement your nutritional efforts, ensuring a holistic approach to optimal mental health and cognitive longevity.

Embrace the journey of feeding your brain with the right nutrients and unlock the full potential of your mind. Let us move forward together, nourishing your brain for a sharper, healthier, and more resilient you.

Next Steps

With a solid understanding of the essential nutrients for brain health, you are now ready to explore **Chapter 3: Building a Brain-Healthy Diet**. In this chapter, we will provide you with practical guidance on designing a balanced diet that prioritizes brain-boosting foods, along with meal plans and recipe ideas to make the transition seamless and enjoyable. Let me know when you are ready to continue, and we will embark on the next phase of your journey towards optimal mental health!

Chapter 3: Building a Brain-Healthy Diet

Welcome to Chapter 3 of **"Nutrition for Neuroplasticity: Feeding Your Brain for Optimal Mental Health."** Now that you understand the fundamental nutrients essential for brain health, it is time to translate that knowledge into actionable steps. This chapter will guide you through designing a balanced, brain-healthy diet that not only supports neuroplasticity but also fits seamlessly into your daily life. We will explore key dietary principles, practical meal planning strategies, delicious recipes, and tips to make your transition to a brain-boosting diet enjoyable and sustainable.

☐ Key Principles of a Brain-Healthy Diet

A brain-healthy diet emphasizes the consumption of nutrient-dense foods that support cognitive function, protect against oxidative stress, and promote overall mental well-being. Here are the core principles to guide your dietary choices:

1. **Variety and Balance:** Incorporate a wide range of foods to ensure you receive all essential nutrients.
2. **Whole Foods Focus:** Prioritize whole, minimally processed foods over refined and packaged options.
3. **Healthy Fats:** Include sources of omega-3 fatty acids and other healthy fats essential for brain health.
4. **Antioxidant-Rich Foods:** Consume plenty of fruits, vegetables, and other foods high in antioxidants to combat oxidative stress.

5. **Adequate Protein:** Ensure sufficient protein intake to support neurotransmitter production and neural repair.
6. **Hydration:** Maintain proper hydration to optimize brain function and cognitive performance.
7. **Limit Harmful Substances:** Reduce or eliminate intake of processed sugars, trans fats, and excessive caffeine or alcohol.

1. Emphasizing Whole, Nutrient-Dense Foods

Whole foods are unprocessed or minimally processed foods that retain their natural nutrients. They form the foundation of a brain-healthy diet by providing essential vitamins, minerals, antioxidants, and healthy fats.

- **Fruits and Vegetables:** Rich in vitamins, minerals, and antioxidants. Aim for a colorful variety to maximize nutrient intake.
- **Whole Grains:** Sources like quinoa, brown rice, and oats provide sustained energy and fiber.
- **Lean Proteins:** Include fish, poultry, legumes, and nuts to support neurotransmitter synthesis.
- **Healthy Fats:** Incorporate sources like avocados, olive oil, and fatty fish to maintain neuronal health.

2. Incorporating Healthy Fats

Healthy fats, particularly omega-3 fatty acids, are vital for brain health. They contribute to the structural integrity of brain cells and facilitate efficient communication between neurons.

- **Omega-3 Rich Foods:**
  - **Fatty Fish:** Salmon, mackerel, sardines, and trout.
  - **Plant-Based Sources:** Flaxseeds, chia seeds, walnuts, and hemp seeds.
  - **Supplements:** Consider fish oil or algal oil supplements if dietary intake is insufficient.
- **Monounsaturated and Polyunsaturated Fats:**
  - **Avocados:** Versatile and rich in monounsaturated fats.
  - **Nuts and Seeds:** Almonds, cashews, and sunflower seeds.
  - **Olive Oil:** Ideal for cooking and dressings, providing heart-healthy fats.

3. Boosting Antioxidant Intake

Antioxidants protect brain cells from oxidative stress, which is linked to cognitive decline and neurodegenerative diseases. Including a variety of antioxidant-rich foods can help maintain brain health.

- **Berries:** Blueberries, strawberries, raspberries, and blackberries are high in flavonoids.
- **Dark Chocolate:** Contains flavonoids and antioxidants; opt for varieties with at least 70% cocoa.
- **Leafy Greens:** Spinach, kale, and Swiss chard offer vitamins A, C, and K.
- **Herbs and Spices:** Turmeric, cinnamon, and oregano provide potent antioxidant properties.

4. Ensuring Adequate Protein Intake

Proteins are the building blocks of neurotransmitters, which are essential for brain communication and mood regulation. Adequate protein intake supports cognitive functions and mental health.

- **Lean Animal Proteins:** Chicken, turkey, and lean cuts of beef or pork.
- **Plant-Based Proteins:** Lentils, chickpeas, black beans, and tofu.
- **Dairy Products:** Greek yogurt, cottage cheese, and cheese.
- **Eggs:** A versatile and complete protein source.

5. Maintaining Hydration

Proper hydration is crucial for maintaining optimal brain function. Dehydration can impair cognitive performance, mood, and overall mental clarity.

- **Water:** Aim for at least eight glasses (64 ounces) per day, adjusting based on activity level and climate.
- **Herbal Teas:** Green tea and other herbal teas can contribute to hydration while providing additional antioxidants.
- **Hydrating Foods:** Cucumbers, oranges, watermelon, and strawberries have high water content.

Practical Meal Planning Strategies

Designing a brain-healthy diet does not have to be overwhelming. Here are practical strategies to help you create balanced meals that support neuroplasticity:

1. Start with a Solid Foundation: The Plate Method

The plate method is a simple way to ensure balanced meals:

- **Half the Plate:** Fill with non-starchy vegetables and fruits.
- **One-Quarter of the Plate:** Include lean proteins such as fish, poultry, legumes, or tofu.
- **One-Quarter of the Plate:** Add whole grains like quinoa, brown rice, or whole wheat bread.
- **Healthy Fats:** Incorporate sources like olive oil, avocado, or a handful of nuts.

2. Plan Ahead with Weekly Meal Prep

Meal prepping can save time and ensure you stick to your brain-healthy diet:

- **Batch Cooking:** Prepare large quantities of staples like quinoa, roasted vegetables, and grilled chicken.
- **Portion Control:** Divide meals into individual servings to simplify daily meal assembly.
- **Storage Solutions:** Use airtight containers to keep prepped meals fresh throughout the week.

3. Incorporate Variety to Prevent Boredom

Eating a wide range of foods not only ensures a diverse nutrient intake but also keeps your meals interesting:

- **Rotate Proteins:** Alternate between different protein sources such as fish, poultry, legumes, and tofu.

- **Explore New Recipes:** Try new cuisines and recipes that emphasize whole, nutrient-dense ingredients.
- **Seasonal Produce:** Take advantage of seasonal fruits and vegetables for freshness and variety.

Delicious Brain-Boosting Recipes

Here are a few recipes to get you started on your brain-healthy journey. These dishes are not only nutritious but also delicious and easy to prepare.

1. Mediterranean Quinoa Salad

Ingredients:

- One cup quinoa, rinsed
- Two cups water or vegetable broth
- One cup cherry tomatoes, halved

- One cucumber, diced
- 1/2 cup Kalamata olives, pitted and sliced
- 1/4 cup red onion, finely chopped
- 1/4 cup feta cheese, crumbled
- Two tablespoons fresh parsley, chopped
- Three tablespoons olive oil
- Two tablespoons lemon juice
- Salt and pepper to taste

Instructions:

1. **Cook Quinoa:** In a medium saucepan, bring water or vegetable broth to a boil. Add quinoa, reduce heat to low, cover, and simmer for 15 minutes or until the liquid is absorbed. Remove from heat and let sit for 5 minutes, then fluff with a fork.
2. **Prepare Vegetables:** In a large bowl, combine cherry tomatoes, cucumber, olives, red onion, feta cheese, and parsley.

3. **Mix Dressing:** In a small bowl, whisk together olive oil, lemon juice, salt, and pepper.
4. **Combine:** Add cooked quinoa to the vegetable mixture and pour the dressing over the top. Toss to combine.
5. **Serve:** Chill in the refrigerator for at least 30 minutes before serving for flavors to meld.

Benefits:

- High in omega-3s from olives and olive oil.
- Packed with antioxidants from tomatoes and cucumbers.
- Provides complete protein from quinoa.

2. Spinach and Mushroom Omelet

Ingredients:

- Three large eggs
- 1/4 cup spinach, chopped
- 1/4 cup mushrooms, sliced
- One tablespoon olive oil
- Salt and pepper to taste
- Optional: a sprinkle of feta cheese

Instructions:

1. **Prepare Vegetables:** In a non-stick skillet, heat olive oil over medium heat. Add mushrooms and sauté until softened, about 5 minutes. Add spinach and cook until wilted. Remove from skillet and set aside.
2. **Beat Eggs:** In a bowl, whisk eggs with a pinch of salt and pepper.
3. **Cook Omelet:** Pour eggs into the same skillet over medium heat. Let cook for about 1-2 minutes until the edges begin to set.

4. **Add Fillings:** Spoon the sautéed vegetables evenly over one half of the omelet. Sprinkle with feta cheese if desired.
5. **Fold and Serve:** Carefully fold the omelet in half and cook for another minute until fully set. Slide onto a plate and serve warm.

Benefits:

- Rich in B vitamins from spinach and eggs.
- Provides high-quality protein.
- Low in carbohydrates, ideal for sustained energy.

3. Berry and Walnut Yogurt Parfait

Ingredients:

- One cup Greek yogurt

- 1/2 cup mixed berries (blueberries, strawberries, raspberries)
- Two tablespoons walnuts, chopped
- One tablespoon honey or maple syrup
- One teaspoon chia seeds (optional)

Instructions:

1. **Layer Ingredients:** In a glass or bowl, layer half of the Greek yogurt.
2. **Add Berries and Nuts:** Top with half of the mixed berries and walnuts.
3. **Repeat Layers:** Add the remaining yogurt, followed by the rest of the berries and walnuts.
4. **Sweeten and Sprinkle:** Drizzle honey or maple syrup over the top and sprinkle with chia seeds if using.
5. **Serve:** Enjoy immediately or refrigerate for a quick brain-boosting breakfast or snack.

Benefits:

- High in antioxidants from berries.
- Provides omega-3s from walnuts.
- Contains probiotics from Greek yogurt for gut-brain health.

Interactive Element: Meal Planning Worksheet

Meal Planning Worksheet

Use this worksheet to plan your weekly brain-healthy meals, ensuring you incorporate essential nutrients to support neuroplasticity.

Day	Breakfast	Lunch	Dinner	Snacks	Notes/Adjustments
Monday	Spinach	Mediter	Baked	Berry	Try

Day	Breakfast	Lunch	Dinner	Snacks	Notes/Adjustments
	and Mushroom Omelet	ranean Quinoa Salad	Salmon with Veggies	and Walnut Yogurt Parfait	adding chia seeds to parfait
Tuesday	Greek Yogurt with Berries	Lentil and Vegetable Soup	Chicken Stir-Fry with Brown Rice	Apple slices with almond butter	Swap quinoa for brown rice
Wednesday	Avocado Toast with Eggs	Kale and Chickpea Salad	Shrimp and Broccoli Pasta	Dark Chocolate and Walnuts	Use whole grain bread for toast
Thursday	Smoothie with Flaxsee	Turkey and Avocad	Tofu and Vegetab	Carrot sticks with	Add turmeric to curry

Day	Breakfast	Lunch	Dinner	Snacks	Notes/Adjustments
	ds	o Wrap	le Curry	hummus	
Friday	Overnight Oats with Berries	Quinoa and Black Bean Bowl	Grilled Steak with Sweet Potatoes	Mixed Nuts and Berries	Use lean cuts of steak
Saturday	Berry and Walnut Yogurt Parfait	Spinach and Feta Stuffed Chicken	Vegetable and Lentil Stew	Fresh Fruit Salad	Include a variety of berries
Sunday	Scrambled Eggs with Veggies	Mediterranean Quinoa Salad	Baked Cod with Asparagus	Greek Yogurt with Honey	Prepare extra quinoa for Monday

Instructions:

1. **Plan Your Meals:** Fill in each meal slot with a balanced, nutrient-dense option.
2. **Ensure Variety:** Incorporate different proteins, vegetables, and grains throughout the week.
3. **Track Nutrient Intake:** Use the meal plans to ensure you are meeting your daily nutrient goals.
4. **Adjust as Needed:** Modify recipes and meal choices based on your preferences and dietary needs.

Personal Anecdote: Emma's Transition to a Brain-Healthy Diet

Emma, a 30-year-old software developer, often felt mentally fatigued and struggled with maintaining focus during her long workdays. Determined to enhance her cognitive performance, Emma decided to overhaul her diet based on the principles outlined in this book. She began by incorporating more omega-3-rich foods like salmon and walnuts into her meals and added a variety of antioxidant-rich berries to her snacks. Emma also started planning her meals weekly, using the Meal Planning Worksheet to ensure she included all essential nutrients.

Within a few months, Emma noticed a remarkable improvement in her mental clarity and focus. Her ability to retain information and solve complex problems enhanced significantly, and she felt more energized throughout the day. By building a brain-healthy diet, Emma not only boosted her cognitive performance but also enjoyed a more vibrant and balanced lifestyle.

Expert Insight: Dr. Laura Mitchell on Designing a Brain-Healthy Diet

"Designing a brain-healthy diet is about making intentional choices that support cognitive function and overall mental well-being. By prioritizing whole, nutrient-dense foods and ensuring a balanced intake of essential nutrients, individuals can significantly enhance their brain health and neuroplasticity. Practical meal planning and incorporating a variety of brain-boosting foods make this approach both effective and sustainable."
— **Dr. Laura Mitchell**, Nutritionist and Cognitive Health Specialist

Interactive Element: Brain-Healthy Grocery List

Brain-Healthy Grocery List

Use this list to stock your pantry and fridge with brain-boosting essentials.

Category	Items
Fruits	Blueberries, strawberries, raspberries, oranges
Vegetables	Spinach, kale, broccoli, bell peppers, sweet potatoes
Whole Grains	Quinoa, brown rice, whole wheat bread, oats
Proteins	Salmon, chicken breast, tofu, lentils, eggs
Healthy Fats	Avocados, walnuts, olive oil, flaxseeds, chia seeds
Dairy	Greek yogurt, cottage cheese, feta cheese
Nuts and Seeds	Almonds, pecans, sunflower seeds, chia seeds
Herbs and Spices	Turmeric, cinnamon, oregano, black pepper
Beverages	Green tea, herbal teas, water
Others	Dark chocolate (70% cocoa or

Category	Items
	higher), honey or maple syrup

Instructions:

1. **Review Your Meal Plans:** Refer to your Meal Planning Worksheet to identify the necessary ingredients.
2. **Organized by Category:** Use the categories to streamline your grocery shopping and ensure you do not miss any brain-boosting foods.
3. **Shop Weekly:** Plan a weekly grocery trip to keep your kitchen stocked with fresh, nutrient-dense foods.
4. **Prepare Ahead:** Consider prepping certain items in advance, such as chopping vegetables or cooking grains, to save time during busy days.

Conclusion

Building a brain-healthy diet is a proactive step toward enhancing your cognitive function, emotional resilience, and overall mental well-being. By embracing the key principles of variety, whole foods, healthy fats, antioxidants, adequate protein, and proper hydration, you lay a solid foundation for supporting neuroplasticity. Practical meal planning, creative recipes, and consistent dietary habits ensure that your journey towards optimal brain health is both enjoyable and sustainable.

In the next chapter, **"Lifestyle Factors and Brain Health,"** we will explore how beyond nutrition, other lifestyle choices like exercise, sleep, and stress management contribute to a holistic approach to brain wellness. You will learn how to integrate these elements seamlessly with your brain-healthy diet to maximize your neuroplasticity and overall mental health.

Embrace the power of mindful nutrition and take charge of your brain health today. Your mind is a powerful tool—fuel it with the right nutrients and watch it flourish.

Chapter 4: Creating Synergy: Combining Nutrition with Lifestyle Habits

Welcome to Chapter 4 of **"Nutrition for Neuroplasticity: Feeding Your Brain for Optimal Mental Health."** Up to this point, we have explored the foundational science of neuroplasticity and identified the essential nutrients that support brain health. Now, it is time to take a holistic approach by integrating these nutritional strategies with other vital lifestyle habits. By creating synergy between your diet, physical activity, sleep, and stress management practices, you can significantly enhance your brain's adaptability, resilience, and overall mental well-being.

☐ The Power of Synergy in Brain Health

Synergy occurs when different elements work together to produce a combined effect greater than the sum of their individual effects. In the context of brain health, combining proper nutrition with other healthy lifestyle habits amplifies the benefits each practice offers. This holistic approach ensures that all aspects of your well-being are addressed, fostering an environment where neuroplasticity can thrive.

Key Benefits of Synergy:

- **Enhanced Cognitive Function:** Improved memory, focus, and problem-solving abilities.
- **Increased Emotional Resilience:** Better management of stress, anxiety, and mood swings.
- **Optimized Physical Health:** Stronger immune system, increased energy levels, and reduced risk of chronic diseases.

- **Sustainable Well-Being:** Long-term maintenance of mental and physical health through balanced habits.

1. Integrating Physical Activity

Physical activity is a cornerstone of a brain-healthy lifestyle. Regular exercise not only supports cardiovascular health but also promotes neurogenesis and synaptic plasticity, enhancing cognitive functions and emotional stability.

Benefits of Physical Activity for the Brain:

- **Increases Blood Flow:** Enhances oxygen and nutrient delivery to brain cells.
- **Promotes Neurogenesis:** Stimulates the growth of new neurons, particularly in the hippocampus.

- **Releases Neurotrophic Factors:** Supports neuron survival and growth.
- **Reduces Inflammation:** Lowers levels of inflammatory markers that can impair brain function.

Types of Exercise to Boost Neuroplasticity:

- **Aerobic Exercise:** Activities like running, swimming, and cycling improve cardiovascular health and increase blood flow to the brain.
- **Strength Training:** Builds muscle mass and bone density while also supporting brain health through hormonal balance.
- **Mind-Body Exercises:** Practices such as yoga and tai chi combine physical movement with mindfulness, enhancing both physical and mental well-being.

- **High-Intensity Interval Training (HIIT):** Alternating between intense bursts of activity and periods of rest can improve cognitive flexibility and executive function.

Practical Tips for Incorporating Exercise:

- **Find Activities You Enjoy:** Choose exercises that you find fun and engaging to ensure consistency.
- **Set Realistic Goals:** Start with manageable goals and gradually increase intensity and duration.
- **Schedule Regular Workouts:** Incorporate exercise into your daily routine, treating it as a non-negotiable appointment.
- **Combine with Nutrition:** Fuel your workouts with brain-healthy foods to maximize performance and recovery.

Personal Anecdote: Michael's Transformation Through Exercise

Michael, a 45-year-old accountant, struggled with chronic stress and declining cognitive function due to long hours at his desk. Determined to improve his mental health, he began incorporating regular aerobic exercise and yoga into his routine. Coupled with a brain-healthy diet rich in omega-3s and antioxidants, Michael experienced enhanced memory, reduced stress levels, and increased overall energy. This holistic approach not only revitalized his mind but also improved his physical health, demonstrating the powerful synergy between nutrition and exercise.

Expert Insight: Dr. Laura Mitchell on Exercise and Neuroplasticity

"Physical activity is indispensable for brain health. Regular exercise stimulates the production of

2. Prioritizing Quality Sleep

Sleep is a fundamental aspect of brain health, playing a critical role in memory consolidation, emotional regulation, and overall cognitive function. Adequate sleep supports neuroplasticity by allowing the brain to repair and reorganize itself.

Benefits of Quality Sleep for the Brain:

- **Memory Consolidation:** Strengthens neural connections formed during the day.
- **Emotional Regulation:** Helps manage stress and maintain emotional balance.
- **Cognitive Function:** Enhances attention, problem-solving, and decision-making skills.
- **Detoxification:** Facilitates the removal of metabolic waste products from the brain.

Strategies for Improving Sleep Quality:

- **Establish a Consistent Sleep Schedule:** Go to bed and wake up at the same time every day, even on weekends.
- **Create a Relaxing Bedtime Routine:** Engage in calming activities such as reading, meditation, or gentle stretching before bed.
- **Optimize Sleep Environment:** Ensure your bedroom is cool, dark, and quiet. Invest in a comfortable mattress and pillows.

- **Limit Exposure to Screens:** Reduce blue light exposure from phones, tablets, and computers at least an hour before bedtime.
- **Mind Your Diet:** Avoid heavy meals, caffeine, and alcohol close to bedtime. Incorporate sleep-promoting foods like cherries, almonds, and herbal teas.

Personal Anecdote: Emma's Sleep Overhaul

Emma, a 32-year-old graphic designer, frequently experienced insomnia and daytime fatigue, which negatively impacted her work and personal life. After consulting with a sleep specialist, Emma implemented a consistent sleep schedule, created a calming bedtime routine, and adjusted her diet to include more sleep-friendly foods. Within a few weeks, Emma noticed significant improvements in her sleep quality, waking up refreshed and alert. The combination of better sleep and a brain-healthy diet enhanced her cognitive performance and emotional well-being.

Expert Insight: Dr. Rebecca White on Sleep and Cognitive Health

"Quality sleep is essential for neuroplasticity. During sleep, the brain consolidates memories and repairs neural connections. A diet rich in tryptophan, magnesium, and antioxidants can support better sleep quality, thereby enhancing overall brain function and mental health."
— **Dr. Rebecca White**, Psychiatrist and Sleep Researcher

3. Effective Stress Management

Chronic stress can have detrimental effects on the brain, impairing neuroplasticity and increasing the risk of mental health disorders. Implementing effective stress management techniques is crucial for maintaining a healthy, adaptable brain.

Impact of Stress on the Brain:

- **Hippocampal Atrophy:** Chronic stress can shrink the hippocampus, a region critical for memory and learning.
- **Reduced Neurogenesis:** Inhibits the growth of new neurons, limiting the brain's ability to adapt and recover.
- **Impaired Synaptic Plasticity:** Hinders the brain's capacity to form and strengthen neural connections.
- **Increased Inflammation:** Promotes inflammatory processes that can damage brain cells and impair cognitive function.

Stress Management Techniques:

- **Mindfulness Meditation:** Practices that cultivate present-moment awareness can reduce stress and enhance emotional regulation.
- **Deep Breathing Exercises:** Techniques like diaphragmatic breathing and box breathing help activate the parasympathetic nervous system, promoting relaxation.
- **Physical Activity:** Regular exercise serves as a natural stress reliever by releasing endorphins and reducing cortisol levels.
- **Time Management:** Organizing tasks and setting priorities can alleviate the pressure of overwhelming responsibilities.
- **Social Support:** Building strong relationships and seeking support from friends and family can buffer against stress.

Practical Tips for Managing Stress:

- **Daily Meditation:** Incorporate at least 10 minutes of mindfulness meditation into your daily routine.
- **Scheduled Breaks:** Take regular breaks throughout the day to rest and recharge.
- **Journaling:** Reflect on your thoughts and emotions to gain perspective and identify stressors.
- **Hobbies and Leisure:** Engage in activities that bring you joy and relaxation, such as reading, painting, or gardening.
- **Professional Help:** Seek guidance from a therapist or counselor if stress becomes unmanageable.

Personal Anecdote: John's Stress Reduction Journey

John, a 40-year-old IT manager, faced high levels of stress due to demanding projects and long working hours. He began practicing mindfulness meditation and incorporated regular exercise into his routine. Additionally, John adopted a brain-healthy diet rich in omega-3s and antioxidants to support his mental resilience. Over time, John experienced reduced stress levels, improved mood, and enhanced cognitive function. These changes not only boosted his professional performance but also enriched his personal life.

Expert Insight: Dr. Samuel Green on Stress and Neuroplasticity

"Chronic stress impairs neuroplasticity and can lead to cognitive decline and emotional instability. Integrating stress management techniques with a nutrient-rich diet creates a protective environment for the brain, fostering resilience and enhancing its

4. Optimizing Gut Health

Emerging research highlights the significant connection between gut health and brain function, often referred to as the **gut-brain axis**. A healthy gut microbiome influences neuroplasticity, mood regulation, and cognitive performance.

The Gut-Brain Connection:

- **Neurotransmitter Production:** Gut bacteria produce neurotransmitters like serotonin and dopamine, which regulate mood and cognition.

- **Immune System Regulation:** A balanced gut microbiome helps modulate the immune system, reducing inflammation that can affect the brain.
- **Nutrient Absorption:** Efficient nutrient absorption supports overall brain health and function.

Foods That Promote Gut Health:

- **Probiotics:** Yogurt, kefir, sauerkraut, kimchi, and other fermented foods introduce beneficial bacteria to the gut.
- **Prebiotics:** Foods like garlic, onions, bananas, asparagus, and whole grains feed and sustain beneficial gut bacteria.
- **Fiber-Rich Foods:** Fruits, vegetables, legumes, and whole grains support a healthy digestive system.

- **Polyphenol-Rich Foods:** Berries, green tea, dark chocolate, and red wine promote the growth of beneficial gut bacteria.

Practical Ways to Support Gut Health:

- **Incorporate Fermented Foods:** Add yogurt or kefir to your breakfast and include fermented vegetables in your meals.
- **Eat a Variety of Plant-Based Foods:** Ensure a diverse intake of fruits, vegetables, and whole grains to nourish your gut microbiome.
- **Stay Hydrated:** Adequate water intake supports digestion and nutrient absorption.
- **Limit Processed Foods:** Reduce consumption of high-sugar and high-fat processed foods that can disrupt gut bacteria balance.

Personal Anecdote: Lisa's Gut Health Transformation

Lisa, a 29-year-old marketing professional, struggled with digestive issues and frequent mood swings. After consulting with a nutritionist, she began incorporating probiotic-rich foods like yogurt and sauerkraut into her diet and increased her intake of prebiotic foods such as garlic and bananas. Additionally, Lisa focused on eating more fiber-rich vegetables and whole grains. Within a few months, Lisa experienced improved digestion, more stable moods, and enhanced cognitive clarity. Her journey underscores the importance of gut health in supporting overall brain function and mental well-being.

Expert Insight: Dr. Emma Stone on the Gut-Brain Axis

"The gut microbiome plays a pivotal role in brain health through the gut-brain axis. By fostering a healthy gut environment with probiotics, prebiotics, and fiber-rich foods, individuals can enhance

neuroplasticity, stabilize mood, and improve cognitive function. A balanced diet is essential for maintaining both gut and brain health."
— **Dr. Emma Stone**, Gastroenterologist and Neuroscience Researcher

---

5. Mindful Eating Practices

Mindful eating is the practice of paying full attention to the experience of eating and drinking, both inside and outside the body. This practice not only enhances the enjoyment of food but also supports better digestion, nutrient absorption, and mental clarity.

Benefits of Mindful Eating:

- **Improved Digestion:** Paying attention to the eating process can enhance digestive efficiency.
- **Better Nutrient Absorption:** Mindful eating allows your body to fully process and absorb nutrients from food.
- **Weight Management:** Increases awareness of hunger and fullness cues, preventing overeating.
- **Enhanced Enjoyment:** Heightens the sensory experience of eating, making meals more satisfying.
- **Reduced Stress:** Creates a calming routine that can lower stress levels associated with eating.

Techniques for Practicing Mindful Eating:

- **Slow Down:** Take your time to chew each bite thoroughly and savor the flavors.

- **Eliminate Distractions:** Eat without distractions such as TV, smartphones, or computers to fully engage with your meal.
- **Engage Your Senses:** Notice the colors, textures, smells, and tastes of your food.
- **Listen to Your Body:** Pay attention to your hunger and fullness signals to avoid overeating.
- **Express Gratitude:** Take a moment to appreciate the effort and resources that went into preparing your meal.

Practical Tips for Incorporating Mindful Eating:

- **Set the Table:** Create a pleasant eating environment to enhance the meal experience.
- **Portion Control:** Serve smaller portions to prevent overeating and allow for mindful consumption.

- **Focus on Quality:** Choose high-quality, nutrient-dense foods that nourish your body and mind.
- **Eat Regularly:** Maintain consistent mealtimes to regulate hunger and prevent binge eating.
- **Reflect Post-Meal:** Take a few minutes after eating to reflect on how the meal made you feel physically and emotionally.

Personal Anecdote: Mark's Journey to Mindful Eating

Mark, a 40-year-old entrepreneur, often rushed through meals while juggling multiple tasks, leading to poor digestion and weight gain. By adopting mindful eating practices, such as eating without distractions and savoring each bite, Mark improved his digestion, stabilized his weight, and felt more satisfied after meals. This shift not only enhanced his physical health but also provided him with mental clarity and reduced stress levels, illustrating the profound impact of mindful eating on overall well-being.

Expert Insight: Dr. Laura Bennett on Mindful Eating and Brain Health

"Mindful eating is a powerful tool for enhancing both physical and mental health. By paying full attention to the eating experience, individuals can improve digestion, optimize nutrient absorption, and foster a healthier relationship with food. This practice supports neuroplasticity by reducing stress and promoting emotional balance."
— **Dr. Laura Bennett**, Clinical Psychologist and Nutritionist

Interactive Element: Lifestyle Synergy Planner

Lifestyle Synergy Planner

Use this planner to integrate nutrition with other healthy lifestyle habits, creating a harmonious routine that supports neuroplasticity and overall brain health.

Day	Nutrition Focus	Exercise Activity	Sleep Goal	Stress Management Technique	Notes/Adjustments
Monday	Omega-3-rich meals	30-minute brisk walk	8 hours of sleep	10 minutes of meditation	Add chia seeds to breakfast
Tuesda	Antioxi	Yoga	Consis	Deep	Include

Day	Nutrition Focus	Exercise Activity	Sleep Goal	Stress Management Technique	Notes/Adjustments
y	dant-packed foods	session	tent bedtime	breathing exercises	berries in snacks
Wednesday	B vitamin-rich diet	Strength training	Power nap (20 mins)	Journaling	Prepare a spinach and mushroom omelet
Thursday	Vitamin D intake	Mindful walking	Relaxing bedtime routine	Progressive muscle relaxation	Increase sun exposure
Friday	Polyphenol-rich	HIIT workout	8 hours	Listen to calming	Add turmeric to

Day	Nutrition Focus	Exercise Activity	Sleep Goal	Stress Management Technique	Notes/Adjustments
	foods	ut	of sleep	music	dinner
Saturday	Probiotic and prebiotic foods	Dance class	Early bedtime	Socialize with friends	Try a new fermented recipe
Sunday	Balanced whole foods	Rest day or light stretching	Plan upcoming week	Reflect on the week	Meal prep for Monday

Instructions:

1. **Plan Your Day:** Fill in each section with specific activities and goals.
2. **Track Progress:** Mark off completed tasks and note any observations or adjustments needed.
3. **Reflect Weekly:** At the end of each week, review your planner to assess what is working and make necessary changes for the following week.

Conclusion

Creating synergy between nutrition and other healthy lifestyle habits is essential for maximizing the benefits of neuroplasticity and achieving optimal mental health. By integrating a brain-healthy diet with regular physical activity, quality sleep, effective stress management, and mindful eating practices, you establish a comprehensive approach to brain wellness. This holistic strategy not only supports the brain's ability to adapt and thrive but also fosters a balanced and fulfilling life.

In the chapters that follow, we will delve deeper into specific meal plans, recipes, and advanced strategies to further enhance your brain health. You will also explore how to sustain these healthy habits long-term, ensuring that your journey towards optimal mental health is both effective and enduring.

Embrace the power of synergy in your lifestyle and watch as your brain and overall well-being flourish. Together, let us create a harmonious routine that nourishes your mind, body, and soul.

Chapter 6: Reducing Stress Through Mindful Movement

Welcome to Chapter 6 of **"Nutrition for Neuroplasticity: Feeding Your Brain for Optimal Mental Health."** As we navigate the complexities of modern life, stress has become an almost inevitable part of our daily existence. Chronic stress not only hampers our mental and physical health but also impairs the brain's ability to adapt and grow through neuroplasticity. Fortunately, mindful movement offers a powerful, holistic approach to managing and reducing stress, fostering a resilient and adaptable mind.

Understanding the Impact of Stress on the Brain

Before diving into mindful movement techniques, it is essential to comprehend how stress affects our brain and overall well-being.

The Physiology of Stress

When we encounter a stressor, our body activates the **fight-or-flight response**, releasing hormones like cortisol and adrenaline. While this response is beneficial for short-term survival, prolonged exposure to stress hormones can lead to detrimental effects:

- **Hippocampal Atrophy:** Chronic stress can shrink the hippocampus, a region crucial for memory and learning.
- **Prefrontal Cortex Impairment:** Reduced function in the prefrontal cortex affects decision-making, attention, and self-control.
- **Amygdala Hyperactivity:** An overactive amygdala heightens anxiety and fear responses.
- **Neuroinflammation:** Persistent stress promotes inflammation in the brain, contributing to cognitive decline and mood disorders.

Neuroplasticity and Stress

Stress inhibits neuroplasticity by disrupting the formation of new neural connections and impairing the brain's ability to reorganize itself. This can lead to difficulties in learning, memory retention, and emotional regulation. However, by incorporating mindful movement into your routine, you can counteract these effects and support a healthier, more adaptable brain.

1. The Role of Mindful Movement in Stress Reduction

Mindful movement integrates physical activity with mindfulness practices, creating a synergistic effect that enhances both mental and physical well-being. Unlike traditional exercise, mindful movement emphasizes awareness, breath control, and intentionality, which are pivotal in managing stress.

Benefits of Mindful Movement:

- **Reduces Cortisol Levels:** Lowers the body's stress hormone, promoting relaxation.

- **Enhances Endorphin Production:** Boosts mood and alleviates feelings of anxiety and depression.
- **Improves Sleep Quality:** Facilitates deeper, more restorative sleep.
- **Increases Mindfulness:** Enhances present-moment awareness, reducing rumination and worry.
- **Promotes Physical Health:** Strengthens muscles, improves flexibility, and boosts cardiovascular health.

2. Types of Mindful Movement Practices for Stress Reduction

Several mindful movement practices have been scientifically proven to reduce stress and support neuroplasticity. Here are some of the most effective ones:

a. Yoga

Yoga combines physical postures, breath control, and meditation, making it a comprehensive practice for stress management.

- **Hatha Yoga:** Focuses on physical postures and breath control, promoting relaxation and flexibility.
- **Vinyasa Yoga:** Involves fluid movements synchronized with breathing, enhancing cardiovascular health and mental focus.
- **Restorative Yoga:** Utilizes props to support the body in passive poses, inducing deep relaxation and stress relief.

Personal Anecdote: Sarah's Journey with Yoga
Sarah, a 34-year-old marketing executive, found herself overwhelmed by the demands of her high-stress job. Incorporating regular yoga practice into her

routine, she experienced significant reductions in anxiety and improved her ability to manage stress. The combination of physical movement and mindfulness allowed Sarah to cultivate a sense of calm and balance, enhancing both her professional and personal life.

b. Tai Chi

Tai Chi is a form of martial arts characterized by slow, deliberate movements and deep breathing, promoting mental clarity and physical relaxation.

- **Benefits:** Enhances balance, reduces stress, improves circulation, and fosters a meditative state.

Case Study: John's Transformation with Tai Chi
John, a 50-year-old teacher, struggled with chronic stress and high blood pressure. After adopting Tai

Chi, he noticed improvements in his blood pressure levels and a marked decrease in stress. The meditative movements helped John achieve a state of mental tranquility, allowing him to navigate his responsibilities with greater ease and composure.

c. Mindful Walking

Mindful walking involves paying full attention to the act of walking, focusing on each step, breath, and sensory experience.

- **Benefits:** Clears the mind, reduces stress, enhances mood, and increases physical activity.

Personal Anecdote: Emily's Mindful Walks Emily, a 28-year-old graphic designer, incorporated mindful walking into her daily routine to combat work-related stress. During her walks, she focused on her breath and the sensations of each step, which helped her release tension and gain mental clarity. This practice not only alleviated her stress but also sparked creativity in her work.

d. Dance Therapy

Dance therapy uses movement to express emotions and reduce stress, combining physical activity with creative expression.

- **Benefits:** Boosts mood, reduces anxiety, improves body image, and fosters social connections.

Case Study: Michael's Healing Through Dance
Michael, a 42-year-old engineer, turned to dance therapy after experiencing burnout. The expressive movements allowed him to process emotions and release built-up stress. Regular dance sessions

revitalized his spirit, improved his mental health, and enhanced his ability to cope with workplace pressures.

3. Creating a Mindful Movement Routine

Establishing a consistent mindful movement routine is key to reaping its stress-reducing benefits. Here is how to create an effective routine tailored to your lifestyle:

a. Start Small and Build Gradually

- **Begin with Short Sessions:** Start with 10-15 minutes of mindful movement each day, gradually increasing the duration as you become more comfortable.
- **Choose Enjoyable Practices:** Select activities that you find enjoyable and sustainable to maintain consistency.

b. Integrate Mindfulness Techniques

- **Focus on Breath:** Incorporate deep breathing exercises to enhance relaxation and presence.
- **Stay Present:** Pay attention to your body's sensations and movements, avoiding distractions.

c. Schedule Regular Sessions

- **Consistency is Key:** Allocate specific times each day for mindful movement to establish it as a habit.
- **Flexibility:** Adapt your routine based on your schedule, ensuring it remains manageable and stress-free.

d. Combine with Nutrition

- **Pre-Movement Nutrition:** Consume light, brain-boosting snacks like a handful of nuts or a piece of fruit before your practice.
- **Post-Movement Nutrition:** Refuel with a balanced meal rich in proteins, healthy fats, and complex carbohydrates to support recovery and brain function.

Interactive Element: Weekly Mindful Movement Planner

Weekly Mindful Movement Planner

Use this planner to schedule and track your mindful movement practices each week, ensuring a balanced and consistent approach to stress reduction.

Day	Activity	Duration	Focus Points (Breath, Movement, Awareness)	Completed (✓)
Monday	Yoga	20 mins	Breath control, flexibility	
Tuesday	Tai Chi	30 mins	Slow movements, mental clarity	
Wednesday	Mindful Walking	15 mins	Step awareness, sensory focus	
Thursday	Dance Therapy	25 mins	Expressive movement,	

Day	Activity	Duration	Focus Points (Breath, Movement, Awareness)	Completed (✓)
			emotional release	
Friday	Yoga	20 mins	Breath control, relaxation	
Saturday	Mindful Walking	20 mins	Nature connection, stress relief	
Sunday	Rest or Light Stretching	10 mins	Gentle movement, relaxation	

Instructions:

1. **Select Activities:** Choose a variety of mindful movement practices that you enjoy and find beneficial.
2. **Set Durations:** Allocate specific durations based on your schedule and fitness level.
3. **Focus Points:** Note the key focus points to enhance mindfulness during each session.
4. **Track Completion:** Mark each activity as completed to stay accountable and motivated.
5. **Reflect Weekly:** At the end of the week, review your planner to assess your progress and make adjustments as needed.

4. Combining Mindful Movement with Nutrition for Enhanced Stress Reduction

To maximize the stress-reducing benefits of mindful movement, it is essential to align your nutritional intake with your physical activities.

a. Pre-Movement Nutrition Tips

- **Light and Energizing:** Opt for easily digestible foods that provide quick energy without causing discomfort.
- **Examples:** A banana, a handful of almonds, or a small smoothie with berries and spinach.

b. Post-Movement Nutrition Tips

- **Replenish Nutrients:** Consume a balanced meal rich in proteins, healthy fats, and complex carbohydrates to support muscle recovery and brain function.

- **Examples:** Grilled chicken with quinoa and steamed vegetables, or tofu stir-fry with brown rice and mixed greens.

c. Hydration

- **Stay Hydrated:** Drink water before, during, and after your mindful movement practices to maintain optimal brain function and physical performance.
- **Infused Waters:** Enhance hydration with natural flavors by adding slices of lemon, cucumber, or mint.

5. Overcoming Common Challenges

Incorporating mindful movement into your routine can present challenges. Here are strategies to overcome them:

a. Lack of Time

- **Short Sessions:** Opt for shorter, more frequent sessions throughout the day.
- **Combine Activities:** Integrate mindful movement with daily tasks, such as stretching while watching TV or walking during phone calls.

b. Motivation and Consistency

- **Set Goals:** Establish clear, achievable goals to stay motivated.
- **Find a Partner:** Practice with a friend or join a class to enhance accountability.
- **Celebrate Milestones:** Acknowledge and reward yourself for reaching your routine goals.

c. Physical Limitations

- **Adapt Practices:** Modify movements to accommodate any physical limitations or seek alternative activities that suit your needs.
- **Consult Professionals:** Work with a yoga instructor or physical therapist to develop safe and effective practice.

Interactive Element: Stress Reduction Log

Stress Reduction Log

Use this log to track your mindful movement practices and monitor their impact on your stress levels and overall well-being.

Date	Activity	Duration	Stress Level Before (1-10)	Stress Level After (1-10)	Notes/Feelings

Date	Activity	Duration	Stress Level Before (1-10)	Stress Level After (1-10)	Notes/Feelings
2024-05-01	Yoga	20 mins	7	4	Felt more relaxed and focused
2024-05-02	Tai Chi	30 mins	8	3	Enjoyed the slow movements
2024-05-03	Mindful Walking	15 mins	6	2	Clear mind, appreciated nature
2024-05-04	Dance Therapy	25 mins	7	3	Released pent-up emotions
2024-05-05	Yoga	20 mins	5	2	Felt calm and rejuvenated
2024-05-06	Mindful Walkin	20 mins	6	2	Energized and refreshed

Date	Activity	Duration	Stress Level Before (1-10)	Stress Level After (1-10)	Notes/Feelings
2024-05-07	Rest	-	4	4	Rest day, felt balanced

Instructions:

1. **Record Each Session:** After completing a mindful movement practice, fill in the details of your session.
2. **Assess Stress Levels:** Rate your stress before and after the activity to gauge its effectiveness.
3. **Reflect on Feelings:** Note any observations, feelings, or thoughts that arose during and after the practice.

4. **Identify Patterns:** Look for trends in your stress levels and the activities that most effectively reduce stress.
5. **Adjust as Needed:** Use your reflections to tailor your routine for maximum stress reduction benefits.

Conclusion

Reducing stress through mindful movement is a powerful strategy for enhancing neuroplasticity and achieving optimal mental health. By incorporating practices like yoga, tai chi, mindful walking, and dance therapy into your daily routine, you create a harmonious blend of physical activity and mindfulness that effectively manages stress and supports brain health. Coupled with a brain-healthy diet, these mindful movement practices provide a comprehensive approach to fostering a resilient, adaptable, and thriving mind.

Remember, the key to success lies in consistency and intentionality. Start by integrating one mindful movement practice into your routine and gradually build upon it as it becomes a natural part of your day. Celebrate your progress, stay patient with yourself, and embrace the journey toward a healthier, happier, and more resilient you.

In the next chapter, **"Enhancing Emotional Well-Being Through Movement,"** we will explore how specific movement practices can further support your emotional health, building upon the stress-reducing benefits you have cultivated through mindful movement. Let us continue advancing our path to comprehensive brain wellness.

Chapter 7: Enhancing Emotional Well-Being Through Movement

Welcome to Chapter 7 of **"Nutrition for Neuroplasticity: Feeding Your Brain for Optimal Mental Health."** As we continue our journey toward optimal brain health, it is essential to recognize the profound impact that physical movement has on our emotional well-being. Emotions are intricately linked to our physical state, and engaging in mindful movement practices can significantly enhance our mood, reduce anxiety, and foster a positive mental state. This chapter delves into the connection between movement and emotional health, explores various movement practices that uplift the spirit, and provides practical strategies to incorporate these practices into your daily life.

☐ The Connection Between Movement and Emotional Health

Emotional well-being is a cornerstone of overall mental health. Our emotions influence how we think, feel, and behave, and in turn, our physical state can profoundly affect our emotional state. Engaging in regular physical activity not only benefits our bodies but also plays a crucial role in regulating emotions, reducing stress, and enhancing mood.

The Science Behind Movement and Emotions

When we engage in physical activity, our bodies release a cascade of biochemical changes that positively influence our emotional state:

- **Endorphin Release:** Often referred to as "feel-good" hormones, endorphins are released during exercise, creating a sense of euphoria and reducing pain perception.

- **Serotonin and Dopamine:** These neurotransmitters play key roles in mood regulation, motivation, and pleasure. Physical activity increases their levels, combating depression and enhancing mood.
- **Cortisol Reduction:** Exercise helps lower cortisol levels, the primary stress hormone, reducing feelings of stress and anxiety.
- **Neuroplasticity Enhancement:** Regular movement supports the growth of new neural connections, improving cognitive flexibility and emotional resilience.

Key Benefits of Movement for Emotional Well-Being:

- **Mood Enhancement:** Regular physical activity leads to sustained improvements in

mood and decreases symptoms of depression
and anxiety.

- **Stress Reduction:** Movement acts as a natural
stress reliever, helping to calm the mind and
body.
- **Increased Self-Esteem:** Achieving fitness
goals and maintaining a healthy lifestyle
boosts self-confidence and self-worth.
- **Better Sleep:** Physical activity promotes
better sleep quality, which is essential for
emotional regulation and mental health.
- **Social Connection:** Group activities and
classes foster a sense of community and
support, combating feelings of loneliness and
isolation.

1. Types of Movement That Enhance Emotional Well-Being

Different types of physical activities offer unique benefits for emotional health. Here are some of the most effective movement practices for enhancing emotional well-being:

a. Dance Therapy

Dance therapy combines expressive movement with therapeutic techniques to improve emotional and psychological health.

- **Benefits:**
    - **Emotional Expression:** Facilitates the release and processing of emotions.
    - **Stress Relief:** Engaging in dance reduces cortisol levels and promotes relaxation.
    - **Joy and Fun:** The playful nature of dance boosts endorphin levels, enhancing mood.

- Social Interaction: Group dance sessions foster connections and a sense of belonging.

Personal Anecdote: Mia's Healing Through Dance
Mia, a 29-year-old artist, faced severe anxiety and struggled to express her emotions verbally. Joining a dance therapy class provided her with a safe space to move and express her feelings through dance. Over time, Mia experienced significant reductions in anxiety, increased self-awareness, and a renewed sense of joy and creativity. Dance therapy became a vital tool in her emotional healing journey, demonstrating the power of movement in fostering emotional well-being.

b. Yoga for Emotional Balance

Yoga integrates physical postures, breath control, and meditation, creating a holistic practice that nurtures both the body and mind.

- **Benefits:**
  - **Mindfulness and Presence:** Enhances awareness and focus, reducing rumination and negative thought patterns.
  - **Relaxation Response:** Activates the parasympathetic nervous system, promoting relaxation and reducing stress.
  - **Emotional Regulation:** Improves the ability to manage emotions and respond calmly to challenges.
  - **Physical Comfort:** Releases physical tension that often accompanies emotional stress.

Case Study: David's Journey with Yoga David, a 40-year-old software developer, experienced chronic stress and burnout due to long hours at his desk. Incorporating daily yoga practice into his routine helped him manage stress, improve his posture, and enhance his overall emotional resilience. The combination of mindful movement and breathwork provided David with tools to stay calm and focused, even during high-pressure situations.

c. Tai Chi for Mental Clarity

Tai Chi is a form of martial arts characterized by slow, deliberate movements and deep breathing, promoting mental clarity and physical relaxation.

- **Benefits:**
    - **Mental Focus:** Enhances concentration and cognitive function through mindful movements.

- o **Emotional Stability:** Reduces anxiety and promotes a sense of inner peace.
- o **Physical Health:** Improves balance, flexibility, and overall physical health.
- o **Mind-Body Connection:** Fosters a deeper connection between physical movement and mental state.

Personal Story: Laura's Calm Through Tai Chi
Laura, a 35-year-old nurse, turned to Tai Chi to cope with the emotional demands of her job. The slow, flowing movements and meditative aspects of Tai Chi provided her with a sense of calm and mental clarity. Regular practice helped Laura reduce work-related stress, improve her emotional resilience, and maintain a positive outlook despite the challenges of her profession.

d. Aerobic Exercise for Mood Boosting

Aerobic exercises such as running, cycling, and swimming are effective for boosting mood and reducing symptoms of depression and anxiety.

- **Benefits:**
    - **Endorphin Surge:** Promotes feelings of happiness and euphoria.
    - **Stress Relief:** Lowers cortisol levels and reduces overall stress.
    - **Cognitive Function:** Enhances memory, learning, and executive function.
    - **Energy Levels:** Increases overall energy and reduces feelings of fatigue.

Case Study: Alex's Transformation Through Running Alex, a 25-year-old student, battled depression and low energy levels. Taking up running as a form of aerobic exercise helped him experience regular endorphin surges, boosting his mood and energy. The physical activity provided Alex with a sense of accomplishment and improved his mental clarity, contributing to a more positive and proactive mindset.

2. Creating a Mindful Movement Routine for Emotional Well-Being

Establishing a consistent mindful movement routine tailored to your emotional needs is essential for sustaining emotional well-being. Here is how to create an effective routine:

a. Assess Your Needs and Preferences

- **Identify Emotional Goals:** Determine what you want to achieve, such as reducing anxiety, boosting mood, or enhancing emotional resilience.

- **Choose Enjoyable Activities:** Select movement practices that you find enjoyable and engaging to ensure consistency.
- **Consider Your Schedule:** Choose times of day that fit seamlessly into your routine, whether it is morning yoga or evening dance sessions.

b. Structure Your Routine

- **Frequency:** Aim for at least three to five sessions per week to maintain consistency and reap the emotional benefits.
- **Duration:** Start with manageable durations, such as 20-30 minutes per session, and gradually increase as you become more comfortable.
- **Variety:** Incorporate different types of mindful movement to keep your routine

interesting and address various aspects of emotional health.

Sample Weekly Mindful Movement Routine:

Day	Activity	Duration	Focus Points (Breath, Movement, Awareness)	Completed (✓)
Monday	Yoga	30 mins	Breath control, emotional release	
Tuesday	Dance Therapy	25 mins	Expressive movement, joy	
Wednesday	Tai Chi	30 mins	Slow movements	

Day	Activity	Duration	Focus Points (Breath, Movement, Awareness)	Completed (✓)
			, mental clarity	
Thursday	Aerobic Exercise	20 mins	Endorphin release, stress reduction	
Friday	Yoga	30 mins	Mindfulness, relaxation	
Saturday	Mindful Walking	20 mins	Step awareness, sensory focus	
Sunday	Rest or	15 mins	Gentle	

Day	Activity	Duration	Focus Points (Breath, Movement, Awareness)	Completed (✓)
	Light Stretching		movement, relaxation	

c. Incorporate Mindfulness Techniques

- **Focus on Breath:** Use deep breathing to enhance relaxation and presence during movement.
- **Stay Present:** Concentrate on each movement and how your body feels, avoiding distractions.

- **Set Intentions:** Begin each session with a clear intention, such as seeking peace, releasing tension, or cultivating joy.

d. Combine with Emotional Nutrition

- **Pre-Movement Snacks:** Consume light, brain-boosting snacks like a handful of nuts or a piece of fruit before your practice.
- **Post-Movement Meals:** Refuel with balanced meals rich in proteins, healthy fats, and complex carbohydrates to support emotional resilience and brain function.

3. Overcoming Common Challenges in Mindful Movement

Implementing a mindful movement routine can present challenges. Here are strategies to overcome them:

a. Time Constraints

- **Short Sessions:** Opt for shorter, more frequent sessions if you have a busy schedule.
- **Integrate into Daily Tasks:** Incorporate mindful movements into daily activities, such as stretching during TV commercials or practicing deep breathing while commuting.

b. Lack of Motivation

- **Set Clear Goals:** Define your emotional well-being goals to stay focused and motivated.
- **Find a Partner:** Practice with a friend or join a class to enhance accountability and enjoyment.
- **Celebrate Progress:** Acknowledge and celebrate small victories to maintain motivation.

c. Physical Limitations

- **Adapt Practices:** Modify movements to accommodate any physical limitations or seek alternative activities that suit your needs.
- **Consult Professionals:** Work with a yoga instructor, dance therapist, or physical therapist to develop a safe and effective practice.

Interactive Element: Emotional Movement Journal

Emotional Movement Journal

Use this journal to track your mindful movement practices and monitor their impact on your emotional well-being.

Date	Activity	Duration	Mood Before (1-10)	Mood After (1-10)	Emotions Experienced	Notes/Observations
2024-05-01	Yoga	30 mins	5	8	Calm, Relaxed	Felt more centered after session
2024-05-02	Dance Therapy	25 mins	6	9	Joyful, Energized	Enjoyed the music and movement
2024-05-03	Tai Chi	30 mins	7	8	Peaceful, Focused	Found the movements soothing
2024-05-	Aerobic	20 mins	4	7	Happy, Refreshe	Endorphin boost felt

Date	Activity	Duration	Mood Before (1-10)	Mood After (1-10)	Emotions Experienced	Notes/Observations
05-04	Exercise				d	great
2024-05-05	Yoga	30 mins	6	8	Relaxed, Content	Deep breathing was beneficial
2024-05-06	Mindful Walking	20 mins	5	7	Clear-minded	Enjoyed being outdoors
2024-05-07	Rest	-	7	7	Neutral	Rest day, felt balanced

Instructions:

1. **Record Each Session:** After completing a mindful movement practice, fill in the details of your session.
2. **Assess Mood:** Rate your mood before and after the activity to gauge its effectiveness.
3. **Identify Emotions:** Note any specific emotions experienced during or after the practice.
4. **Reflect on Observations:** Write down any thoughts, feelings, or insights that arose during the session.
5. **Adjust as Needed:** Use your reflections to tailor your routine for maximum emotional benefits.

4. Combining Movement with Emotional Nutrition

To further enhance emotional well-being through movement, it is essential to align your nutritional intake with your physical practices.

a. Pre-Movement Nutrition for Emotional Support

- **Energizing Snacks:** Choose snacks that provide sustained energy without causing a sugar crash, such as a banana with almond butter or a handful of trail mix.
- **Hydration:** Drink water or herbal teas to stay hydrated, which is crucial for maintaining energy levels and cognitive function.

b. Post-Movement Nutrition for Emotional Recovery

- **Protein-Rich Meals:** Support muscle recovery and neurotransmitter production with lean proteins like chicken, tofu, or legumes.

- **Healthy Fats:** Incorporate sources like avocado, nuts, and olive oil to maintain brain health and emotional balance.
- **Complex Carbohydrates:** Provide sustained energy and enhance mood by including whole grains, sweet potatoes, and vegetables in your meals.

Sample Post-Movement Meal:

- **Grilled Salmon with Quinoa and Steamed Broccoli:** Provides omega-3 fatty acids, complete proteins, and fiber-rich vegetables to support brain function and emotional resilience.

5. Sustaining Your Emotional Well-Being Through Movement

Maintaining emotional well-being through mindful movement requires commitment and adaptability. Here are strategies to sustain your practice:

a. Set Realistic Goals

- **Start Small:** Begin with manageable sessions and gradually increase intensity and duration.
- **Focus on Consistency:** Aim for regular practice rather than perfection, building habits that fit your lifestyle.

b. Stay Inspired

- **Explore Different Practices:** Try various movement forms to find what resonates most with you.
- **Join Communities:** Engage with groups or classes to stay motivated and share experiences.

- **Track Progress:** Use journals and planners to monitor your growth and celebrate milestones.

c. Listen to Your Body and Mind

- **Respect Your Limits:** Avoid pushing yourself too hard and allow for rest when needed.
- **Adjust Practices:** Modify or change activities based on how you feel, ensuring your routine remains enjoyable and effective.

Interactive Element: Emotional Well-Being Tracker

Emotional Well-Being Tracker

Use this tracker to monitor the impact of your mindful movement practices on your emotional health over time.

Week	Number of Sessions	Average Mood Improvement (1-10)	Key Emotional Benefits Achieved	Challenges Faced	Adjustments for Next Week
Week one	5	3	Reduced anxiety, increased joy	Time management	Schedule morning sessions
Week two	6	4	Improved focus, emotional release	Consistency	Set reminders
Week three	7	5	Enhanced mood, better stress management	Physical fatigue	Incorporate more hydration

Week	Number of Sessions	Average Mood Improvement (1-10)	Key Emotional Benefits Achieved	Challenges Faced	Adjustments for Next Week
Week four	6	4	Greater emotional resilience	Lack of variety	Try new movement styles

Instructions:

1. **Record Weekly Data:** Fill in the number of sessions completed, average mood improvement, and key emotional benefits each week.
2. **Identify Challenges:** Note any obstacles that hindered your practice.

3. **Plan Adjustments:** Make necessary changes to your routine to overcome challenges and enhance benefits for the following week.
4. **Reflect on Progress:** Assess how your emotional well-being has improved over time and adjust goals as needed.

Conclusion

Enhancing emotional well-being through mindful movement is a powerful strategy for fostering a resilient and positive mindset. By integrating practices such as dance therapy, yoga, Tai Chi, and aerobic exercise into your routine, you create a dynamic interplay between physical activity and emotional health. These practices not only reduce stress and improve mood but also support the brain's ability to adapt and thrive through neuroplasticity.

Coupled with a brain-healthy diet, mindful movement forms the foundation of a holistic approach to mental health, ensuring that both your mind and body are nourished and supported. Remember, the key to success lies in consistency, enjoyment, and the willingness to adapt your practices to suit your evolving needs.

As you continue on this journey, embrace the transformative power of movement and witness how it elevates your emotional well-being, enriches your mental health, and enhances your overall quality of life. Let movement be your ally in cultivating a happier, healthier, and more resilient you.

In the next chapter, **"Building Resilience Through Mindful Nutrition and Movement,"** we will explore advanced strategies to further strengthen your mental resilience, combining the principles of nutrition and mindful movement to empower you to navigate life's challenges with grace and strength. Let us continue building on the foundation you have established and take the next step toward comprehensive brain wellness.

Chapter 8: Building Resilience Through Mindful Nutrition and Movement

Welcome to Chapter 8 of **"Nutrition for Neuroplasticity: Feeding Your Brain for Optimal Mental Health."** Throughout this book, we have explored the intricate connections between nutrition, neuroplasticity, and various lifestyle habits that support mental health. In this chapter, we delve deeper into the concept of resilience—the ability to adapt, recover, and thrive in the face of adversity. By combining mindful nutrition with purposeful movement, you can significantly enhance your mental resilience, equipping yourself to navigate life's challenges with strength and grace.

☐ Understanding Resilience

Resilience is not an innate trait but a skill that can be developed and strengthened over time. It involves a combination of cognitive, emotional, and physical strategies that help individuals cope with stress, recover from setbacks, and maintain a positive outlook despite difficulties.

The Components of Resilience:

1. **Emotional Regulation:** The ability to manage and respond to emotional experiences in a healthy manner.
2. **Cognitive Flexibility:** The capacity to adapt thinking and behavior in response to changing circumstances.
3. **Social Support:** Building and maintaining strong relationships that provide encouragement and assistance.

4. **Physical Well-Being:** Maintaining a healthy body through nutrition, exercise, and adequate rest.
5. **Purpose and Meaning:** Having clear goals and a sense of purpose that drives motivation and perseverance.

1. The Role of Mindful Nutrition in Building Resilience

Nutrition plays a pivotal role in supporting the brain's ability to adapt and recover. Certain nutrients enhance cognitive function, stabilize mood, and reduce the physiological impacts of stress, all of which contribute to increased resilience.

Key Nutrients for Resilience:

- **Magnesium:** Supports nerve function and reduces anxiety.

- **Vitamin C:** Enhances immune function and lowers cortisol levels.
- **Zinc:** Vital for neurotransmitter production and immune health.
- **Probiotics:** Promote gut health, which is linked to mood regulation.
- **Complex Carbohydrates:** Provide steady energy and support serotonin production.

Practical Ways to Incorporate Resilience-Building Nutrients:

- **Breakfast:** Whole grain oatmeal topped with almonds and blueberries.
- **Lunch:** Spinach and quinoa salad with grilled chicken, avocado, and a citrus vinaigrette.
- **Snacks:** Greek yogurt with a sprinkle of chia seeds and fresh strawberries.
- **Dinner:** Baked salmon with sweet potatoes and steamed broccoli.

- **Hydration:** Infused water with lemon and cucumber slices.

Personal Anecdote: David's Nutritional Transformation

David, a 38-year-old project manager, often felt overwhelmed by work-related stress, leading to burnout and decreased productivity. After consulting with a nutritionist, he revamped his diet to include more magnesium-rich foods like leafy greens and nuts, vitamin C sources such as citrus fruits, and probiotics from yogurt and fermented vegetables. Within three months, David noticed improved mood stability, increased energy levels, and a greater ability to handle stress without feeling drained. His enhanced diet played a crucial role in rebuilding his resilience and overall mental well-being.

Expert Insight: Dr. Amanda Lee on Nutrition and Resilience

"A well-balanced diet is fundamental to building resilience. Nutrient-dense foods provide the necessary support for brain function, emotional regulation, and physical health, all of which are critical components of resilience. By prioritizing mindful nutrition, individuals can strengthen their ability to cope with and recover from life's challenges."
— **Dr. Amanda Lee**, Clinical Nutritionist and Resilience Researcher

---

2. The Power of Movement in Enhancing Resilience

Physical movement not only benefits the body but also fortifies the mind. Regular exercise promotes the release of endorphins, improves sleep quality, and enhances cognitive flexibility—all essential for building resilience.

Types of Movement for Resilience:

- **Strength Training:** Builds physical and mental strength, enhancing confidence.
- **Cardiovascular Exercise:** Improves heart health and reduces anxiety.
- **Mind-Body Practices:** Yoga, Tai Chi, and Pilates foster mental clarity and emotional balance.
- **High-Intensity Interval Training (HIIT):** Boosts resilience by challenging the body and mind through varied intensity.

Practical Ways to Incorporate Resilience-Building Movement:

- **Morning:** Start the day with a 15-minute yoga session to set a positive tone.
- **Afternoon:** Take a brisk 20-minute walk during lunch breaks to clear your mind.
- **Evening:** Engage in strength training exercises three times a week to build physical resilience.
- **Weekly:** Participate in a dance class or Tai Chi session to enhance mental and emotional flexibility.

Case Study: Maria's Resilience Through Strength Training

Maria, a 45-year-old nurse, faced significant emotional strain due to long hours and high-stress environments. She began incorporating strength training into her routine, focusing on compound movements like squats and deadlifts. The physical challenge of lifting weights translated into mental resilience, helping Maria build confidence and manage stress more effectively. Over six months, Maria experienced not only increased physical strength but also improved emotional stability and a stronger sense of self-efficacy.

Expert Insight: Dr. Robert Kim on Movement and Mental Fortitude

"Physical exercise is a powerful tool for building resilience. It not only strengthens the body but also enhances mental fortitude by promoting neuroplasticity, reducing stress hormones, and fostering a sense of accomplishment. Integrating regular movement into one's routine is essential for developing the capacity to withstand and recover from adversity."
— **Dr. Robert Kim**, Sports Psychologist and Movement Therapist

3. Integrating Nutrition and Movement for Maximum Resilience

Combining mindful nutrition with purposeful movement creates a synergistic effect that amplifies the benefits of each practice. Here is how to integrate these elements effectively:

a. Pre-Workout Nutrition for Enhanced Performance and Resilience

- **Balanced Snacks:** Consume a mix of complex carbohydrates and protein to fuel your workouts and support muscle repair.
    - **Examples:** Whole grain toast with peanut butter, a banana with a handful of nuts, or a smoothie with spinach, berries, and protein powder.

- **Hydration:** Drink water or an electrolyte-infused beverage before exercising to maintain optimal hydration levels.

b. Post-Workout Nutrition for Recovery and Mental Clarity

- **Protein-Rich Meals:** Support muscle recovery and neurotransmitter production with lean proteins.
  - **Examples:** Grilled chicken with quinoa and steamed vegetables, tofu stir-fry with brown rice, or a protein-packed salad with beans and avocado.
- **Healthy Fats and Complex Carbohydrates:** Include sources like olive oil, sweet potatoes, and whole grains to replenish energy stores and promote brain health.

c. Timing and Consistency

- **Regular Mealtimes:** Align your meals with your exercise schedule to ensure consistent nutrient intake and energy levels.
- **Consistent Workout Schedule:** Establish a routine that balances different types of movement, ensuring that both your body and mind receive comprehensive support.

d. Mindful Movement Practices Combined with Nutrition

- **Yoga with Hydrating Snacks:** Enjoy a light snack before a yoga session to maintain energy without feeling sluggish.
- **Strength Training with Protein Intake:** Pair strength workouts with a protein-rich meal to maximize muscle repair and cognitive benefits.
- **Cardio with Antioxidant-Rich Foods:** Support cardiovascular health and reduce

oxidative stress by combining aerobic exercise with antioxidant-rich meals.

Personal Anecdote: Lisa's Holistic Approach to Resilience

Lisa, a 32-year-old entrepreneur, sought to enhance her resilience to better manage the demands of her growing business. She adopted a holistic approach by integrating a nutrient-dense diet with a balanced exercise routine. Lisa ensured she consumed omega-3-rich foods like salmon and walnuts to support brain health and paired her strength training sessions with protein-packed meals for optimal recovery. Additionally, she incorporated regular mindfulness practices like meditation and yoga to maintain emotional balance. This comprehensive strategy not only fortified Lisa's mental resilience but also improved her overall productivity and quality of life.

Expert Insight: Dr. Samantha Green on Holistic Resilience

"Building resilience requires a holistic approach that addresses both nutritional and physical aspects of health. By integrating mindful eating with regular movement, individuals can create a robust foundation that supports mental fortitude, emotional stability, and physical well-being. This synergy is essential for developing the capacity to adapt and thrive in the face of adversity."
— **Dr. Samantha Green**, Holistic Nutritionist and Resilience Coach

4. Creating a Resilience-Building Routine

Establishing a consistent routine that combines mindful nutrition, and purposeful movement is key to building resilience. Here is a step-by-step guide to creating your personalized resilience-building routine:

a. Assess Your Current Lifestyle

- **Identify Stressors:** Recognize the primary sources of stress in your life.
- **Evaluate Nutrition:** Assess your current dietary habits and identify areas for improvement.
- **Analyze Physical Activity:** Determine the frequency and type of physical activity you currently engage in.
- **Reflect on Sleep and Recovery:** Evaluate your sleep quality and recovery practices.

b. Set Clear Resilience Goals

- **Define Objectives:** Establish what you want to achieve, such as improved stress

management, enhanced cognitive function, or increased physical strength.
- **Make SMART Goals:** Ensure your goals are Specific, Measurable, Achievable, Relevant, and Time-bound.

c. Design Your Routine

- **Morning:**
    - **Hydration:** Start with a glass of water infused with lemon.
    - **Nutrient-Rich Breakfast:** Include proteins, healthy fats, and complex carbohydrates.
    - **Morning Movement:** Engage in a 15-minute yoga session or a brisk walk.
- **Midday:**
    - **Balanced Lunch:** Incorporate lean proteins, whole grains, and a variety of vegetables.

- o **Mindful Break:** Take a 10-minute mindfulness meditation or deep breathing exercise.
  - o **Physical Activity:** Include a 20-minute strength training or aerobic workout.
- **Evening:**
  - o **Nutritious Dinner:** Focus on a protein-rich meal with healthy fats and fiber.
  - o **Relaxation:** Participate in a calming activity such as Tai Chi or dance therapy.
  - o **Sleep Preparation:** Establish a consistent bedtime routine with relaxation techniques.

d. Monitor and Adjust

- **Track Progress:** Use planners and journals to monitor your adherence to the routine and the impact on your resilience.
- **Reflect Weekly:** Assess what's working and what needs adjustment.
- **Stay Flexible:** Be open to modifying your routine to better suit your evolving needs and circumstances.

Interactive Element: Resilience Routine Planner

Resilience Routine Planner

Use this planner to create and maintain a consistent routine that combines mindful nutrition and purposeful movement, fostering mental resilience and overall well-being.

Time of Day	Activity	Duration	Focus Points (Nutrition, Movement, Mindfulness)	Completed (✓)
Morning	Hydration	5 mins	Rehydrate, vitamin C intake	
Morning	Nutrient-Rich Breakfast	20 mins	Balanced nutrients, brain-boosting foods	
Morning	Yoga/Brisk Walk	15 mins	Flexibility, blood flow, mental clarity	
Midday	Balanced Lunch	30 mins	Protein, fiber,	

Time of Day	Activity	Duration	Focus Points (Nutrition, Movement, Mindfulness)	Completed (✓)
			healthy fats	
Midday	Mindful Break (Meditation)	10 mins	Focus, anxiety reduction	
Midday	Strength Training/Cardio	20 mins	Physical activity, endorphin release	
Evening	Nutritious Dinner	30 mins	Protein, healthy fats, complex carbs	
Evening	Relaxation	25 mins	Emotional	

Time of Day	Activity	Duration	Focus Points (Nutrition, Movement, Mindfulness)	Completed (✓)
g	(Tai Chi/Dance)		release, mental clarity	
Night	Sleep Preparation Routine	15 mins	Relaxation, consistent bedtime	

Instructions:

1. **Fill in Your Planner:** Assign specific activities to different times of the day based on your schedule and preferences.
2. **Track Completion:** Mark each activity as completed to stay accountable and motivated.

3. **Reflect and Adjust:** At the end of each week, review your planner to assess your progress and make necessary adjustments for the following week.

---

5. Sustaining Resilience Through Continuous Practice

Building resilience is an ongoing process that requires dedication and adaptability. Here are strategies to sustain and further enhance your resilience through mindful nutrition and movement:

a. Embrace Lifelong Learning

- **Stay Informed:** Keep up with the latest research on nutrition, neuroplasticity, and resilience to continually refine your practices.

- **Experiment:** Try new foods, recipes, and movement practices to keep your routine exciting and comprehensive.

b. Cultivate a Supportive Environment

- **Social Connections:** Surround yourself with supportive individuals who encourage your resilience-building efforts.
- **Healthy Habits:** Foster an environment that promotes healthy eating and regular physical activity, both at home and in your community.

c. Practice Self-Compassion

- **Be Kind to Yourself:** Acknowledge that building resilience is a journey with ups and downs. Celebrate your progress and learn from setbacks without judgment.

- **Set Realistic Expectations:** Understand that change takes time and effort. Set achievable goals and be patient with your growth.

d. Integrate Mindfulness into Daily Life

- **Continuous Mindfulness:** Incorporate mindfulness into everyday activities, such as eating, walking, and working, to maintain a state of awareness and presence.
- **Regular Reflection:** Take time to reflect on your experiences, emotions, and progress to stay aligned with your resilience goals.

Personal Anecdote: Kevin's Ongoing Resilience Journey

Kevin, a 50-year-old teacher, committed to building resilience through mindful nutrition and movement. Over the years, Kevin consistently followed his resilience routine, integrating new practices like intermittent fasting and Pilates to keep his routine dynamic. He also joined a local yoga community, which provided social support and accountability. Kevin's dedication paid off as he developed a robust ability to handle stress, recover from setbacks, and maintain a positive outlook despite life's challenges. His ongoing journey highlights the importance of continuous practice and adaptability in sustaining resilience.

Expert Insight: Dr. Laura Bennett on Sustaining Resilience

"Resilience is built through consistent, mindful practices that integrate both nutrition and movement. By continuously adapting and evolving your routines, you ensure that your resilience remains strong and capable of withstanding life's inevitable challenges. Embracing a holistic approach fosters a balanced

Interactive Element: Resilience Milestone Tracker

Resilience Milestone Tracker

Use this tracker to celebrate your achievements and monitor your ongoing resilience-building efforts.

Milestone	Date Achieved	Description	Reward/Self-Care Activity
Completed 30-Day Routine	2024-06-01	Successfully followed the resilience routine for 30	Enjoy a spa day or favorite meal

Milestone	Date Achieved	Description	Reward/Self-Care Activity
		days	
Increased Workout Intensity	2024-07-15	Enhanced strength training sessions by ten%	Buy new workout gear
Mastered Mindful Eating	2024-08-10	Consistently practiced mindful eating for 3 months	Take a weekend getaway
Improved Sleep Quality	2024-09-05	Achieved 8 hours of restful sleep consistently	Treat yourself to a new book
Achieved Emotional Goals	2024-10-20	Successfully managed anxiety through	Schedule a fun outing with friends

Milestone	Date Achieved	Description	Reward/Self-Care Activity
		routine	

Instructions:

1. **Set Milestones:** Define key achievements related to your resilience goals.
2. **Track Progress:** Record the date you achieve each milestone and describe the accomplishment.
3. **Reward Yourself:** Assign a self-care activity or reward to celebrate each achievement, reinforcing positive behavior.
4. **Review Regularly:** Periodically assess your milestones to stay motivated and recognize your growth.

Conclusion

Building resilience through mindful nutrition and movement is a transformative journey that empowers you to face life's challenges with strength, adaptability, and grace. By integrating nutrient-dense foods with purposeful physical activity, you create a holistic foundation that supports your brain's ability to adapt and thrive. This synergy not only enhances your cognitive function and emotional well-being but also fosters a resilient mindset capable of overcoming adversity.

Remember, resilience is cultivated through consistent practice and a willingness to embrace change. Start by implementing small, manageable changes to your diet and movement routines, gradually building upon them as they become ingrained in your daily life. Celebrate your progress, stay patient with yourself, and remain committed to your resilience-building journey.

In the next chapter, **"Advanced Strategies for Cognitive Longevity,"** we will explore cutting-edge techniques and emerging research that further enhance brain health and cognitive longevity. From intermittent fasting to advanced supplementation, these strategies will provide you with the tools to maintain a sharp, healthy mind well into the future. Let us continue advancing our path to comprehensive brain wellness and sustained mental excellence.

Chapter 9: Advanced Strategies for Cognitive Longevity

Welcome to Chapter 9 of **"Nutrition for Neuroplasticity: Feeding Your Brain for Optimal Mental Health."** As we approach the culmination of our journey, it is time to delve into advanced strategies that not only support but also enhance cognitive longevity. This chapter explores cutting-edge techniques and emerging research designed to sustain and elevate your brain's performance well into the future. From intermittent fasting and advanced supplementation to cognitive training and lifestyle hacks, these strategies provide a comprehensive toolkit for maintaining a sharp, healthy mind over the long term.

☐ The Quest for Cognitive Longevity

Cognitive longevity refers to the sustained maintenance of cognitive functions—such as memory, attention, and problem-solving—throughout one's lifespan. Achieving cognitive longevity involves a multifaceted approach that combines optimal nutrition, physical activity, mental stimulation, and healthy lifestyle habits. By integrating advanced strategies into your daily routine, you can significantly enhance your brain's resilience, adaptability, and overall performance.

The Importance of Cognitive Longevity:

- **Enhanced Quality of Life:** Maintaining cognitive functions contributes to independence, productivity, and overall well-being in later years.
- **Prevention of Neurodegenerative Diseases:** Strategies that promote cognitive longevity can reduce the risk of conditions like Alzheimer's and Parkinson's.
- **Sustained Mental Clarity:** Ensures ongoing ability to learn, adapt, and engage in meaningful activities.
- **Emotional Stability:** Supports mental health by fostering a sense of purpose and achievement.

1. Intermittent Fasting: Harnessing the Power of Meal Timing

Intermittent fasting (IF) has gained significant attention for its potential benefits in promoting cognitive longevity. By cycling between periods of eating and fasting, IF can enhance brain health through various mechanisms.

Benefits of Intermittent Fasting for the Brain:

- **Autophagy Activation:** Fasting triggers autophagy, a process where the body cleans out damaged cells, including neurons, promoting brain health.
- **Increased Brain-Derived Neurotrophic Factor (BDNF):** IF boosts BDNF levels, which support neuroplasticity and the growth of new neurons.
- **Enhanced Insulin Sensitivity:** Improves glucose metabolism in the brain, reducing the risk of insulin resistance-related cognitive decline.

- **Reduced Inflammation:** Lowers inflammatory markers that can impair brain function and contribute to neurodegenerative diseases.

Popular Intermittent Fasting Protocols:

- **16/8 Method:** Fasting for 16 hours and eating within an 8-hour window each day.
- **5:2 Diet:** Consuming a regular diet for five days and restricting calorie intake to 500-600 calories on two non-consecutive days.
- **Eat-Stop-Eat:** Undertaking a 24-hour fast once or twice a week.

Practical Tips for Implementing Intermittent Fasting:

- **Start Gradually:** Begin with shorter fasting periods, such as 12 hours, and gradually increase as your body adapts.
- **Stay Hydrated:** Drink plenty of water, herbal teas, and black coffee during fasting periods to stay hydrated and curb hunger.
- **Balanced Meals:** Ensure that your eating windows include nutrient-dense foods to provide the necessary vitamins, minerals, and macronutrients.
- **Listen to Your Body:** Pay attention to hunger cues and adjust fasting schedules if you experience adverse effects.

Personal Anecdote: James' Cognitive Boost Through Intermittent Fasting

James, a 45-year-old software developer, struggled with mental fatigue and declining focus. After researching intermittent fasting, he decided to try the

16/8 method, skipping breakfast and consuming his meals between noon and 8 PM. Within a few weeks, James noticed improved mental clarity, increased energy levels, and enhanced concentration at work. By incorporating IF into his routine, James not only boosted his cognitive performance but also achieved better overall health.

Expert Insight: Dr. Elena Martinez on Intermittent Fasting and Brain Health

"Intermittent fasting offers a promising avenue for enhancing cognitive longevity. By promoting autophagy and increasing BDNF levels, IF supports the brain's ability to repair and regenerate. However, it is essential to approach fasting mindfully and ensure that nutritional needs are met during eating periods."

— **Dr. Elena Martinez**, Neuroscientist and Nutrition Specialist

2. Advanced Supplementation: Beyond the Basics

While a balanced diet provides essential nutrients, advanced supplementation can offer targeted support for cognitive longevity. However, it is crucial to approach supplementation with caution and professional guidance.

Key Supplements for Cognitive Longevity:

1. **Omega-3 Fatty Acids (DHA and EPA):**
   - **Role:** Essential for maintaining neuronal membrane fluidity and supporting synaptic plasticity.
   - **Sources:** Fish oil supplements, algal oil (for vegetarians/vegans).

- **Dosage:** 1,000-2,000 mg daily, depending on dietary intake.

2. **Vitamin D3:**
   - **Role:** Supports neuroprotection and the regulation of neurotrophic factors.
   - **Sources:** Vitamin D3 supplements, fortified foods, sunlight exposure.
   - **Dosage:** 2,000 IU daily, adjusted based on blood levels.

3. **Bacopa Monnieri:**
   - **Role:** An adaptogenic herb that enhances memory, learning, and cognitive processing.
   - **Sources:** Herbal supplements.
   - **Dosage:** 300 mg daily standardized to 50% bacosides.

4. **Lion's Mane Mushroom:**
   - **Role:** Promotes neurogenesis and supports brain health by stimulating NGF (nerve growth factor) production.

- o **Sources:** Mushroom extracts and supplements.
- o **Dosage:** 500-1,000 mg daily.

5. **Curcumin:**
   - o **Role:** A potent antioxidant and anti-inflammatory compound that supports brain health and reduces oxidative stress.
   - o **Sources:** Turmeric supplements, especially those formulated with piperine for enhanced absorption.
   - o **Dosage:** 500 mg daily with black pepper extract.

6. **Phosphatidylserine:**
   - o **Role:** A phospholipid that supports cell membrane integrity and cognitive function.
   - o **Sources:** Phosphatidylserine supplements derived from soy or sunflower.

- **Dosage:** 100 mg three times daily.
7. **Nootropics (e.g., L-Theanine, Rhodiola Rosea):**
   - **Role:** Enhance cognitive function, reduce stress, and improve focus.
   - **Sources:** Nootropic blends and individual supplements.
   - **Dosage:** Varies based on specific nootropic and desired effects.

Practical Tips for Safe Supplementation:

- **Consult a Professional:** Always consult with a healthcare provider before starting any new supplement regimen.
- **Quality Matters:** Choose high-quality supplements from reputable brands to ensure purity and efficacy.

- **Start Slowly:** Introduce one supplement at a time to monitor its effects and identify any adverse reactions.
- **Monitor Dosages:** Adhere to recommended dosages and avoid excessive intake, which can lead to toxicity or side effects.
- **Consider Interactions:** Be aware of potential interactions between supplements and any medications you are taking.

Personal Anecdote: Laura's Enhanced Cognitive Function with Supplements

Laura, a 50-year-old teacher, sought to maintain her cognitive sharpness as she approached retirement. After consulting with a nutritionist, she incorporated supplements like Bacopa Monnieri, Lion's Mane, and curcumin into her daily regimen. Over six months, Laura experienced improved memory retention, enhanced focus, and a greater sense of mental clarity.

The targeted supplementation provided the additional support her brain needed to stay resilient and adaptable.

Expert Insight: Dr. Robert Kim on Advanced Supplementation

"Advanced supplementation can play a significant role in supporting cognitive longevity, especially when dietary intake alone may not suffice. However, it is essential to approach supplementation thoughtfully, prioritizing evidence-based nutrients and consulting with healthcare professionals to tailor protocols to individual needs."
— **Dr. Robert Kim**, Clinical Pharmacologist and Supplement Researcher

3. Cognitive Training and Brain Exercises: Stimulating Neuroplasticity

Engaging in cognitive training and brain exercises can significantly enhance neuroplasticity, supporting the brain's ability to adapt and maintain cognitive functions.

Benefits of Cognitive Training:

- **Enhanced Memory:** Improves both short-term and long-term memory retention.
- **Increased Attention and Focus:** Boosts the ability to concentrate and sustain attention.
- **Improved Problem-Solving Skills:** Enhances critical thinking and analytical abilities.
- **Cognitive Flexibility:** Increases adaptability in thinking and responding to new situations.

Effective Cognitive Training Techniques:

1. **Brain Games and Puzzles:**
    o **Examples:** Sudoku, crossword puzzles, memory games, and strategy-based games like chess.
    o **Benefits:** Stimulates various cognitive functions, including memory, problem-solving, and logical reasoning.
2. **Dual N-Back Training:**
    o **Description:** A memory sequence game that challenges working memory and fluid intelligence.
    o **Benefits:** Enhances cognitive control and memory capacity.
3. **Learning a New Skill or Language:**
    o **Examples:** Learning to play a musical instrument, picking up a new language, or mastering a new hobby.

- o **Benefits:** Promotes neurogenesis and strengthens neural connections by engaging multiple brain regions.
4. **Mindfulness and Meditation:**
   - o **Description:** Practices that enhance present-moment awareness and cognitive focus.
   - o **Benefits:** Improves attention, reduces mind-wandering, and supports emotional regulation.
5. **Virtual Reality (VR) Cognitive Training:**
   - o **Description:** Immersive VR programs designed to challenge and stimulate cognitive functions.
   - o **Benefits:** Provides engaging and interactive environments for comprehensive brain stimulation.

Practical Tips for Incorporating Cognitive Training:

- **Consistency is Key:** Engage in cognitive training activities regularly to maximize benefits.
- **Variety Matters:** Mix different types of cognitive exercises to stimulate various brain functions.
- **Challenge Yourself:** Gradually increase the difficulty of tasks to continue promoting neuroplasticity.
- **Track Progress:** Monitor your performance over time to assess improvements and adjust training intensity.

Personal Anecdote: Michael's Cognitive Enhancement Through Learning

Michael, a 60 year-old retiree, wanted to keep his mind sharp after leaving his career as an engineer. He decided to learn Spanish and took up playing the piano. These new skills challenged his brain, leading to improved memory, enhanced problem-solving abilities, and a greater sense of accomplishment. Michael's dedication to continuous learning exemplifies how cognitive training can support neuroplasticity and cognitive longevity.

Expert Insight: Dr. Samantha Green on Cognitive Training

"Cognitive training is a powerful tool for enhancing neuroplasticity and maintaining cognitive functions as we age. By consistently challenging the brain with diverse and progressively difficult tasks, individuals can support their brain's adaptability and resilience, ultimately contributing to cognitive longevity."
— **Dr. Samantha Green**, Cognitive Neuroscientist and Brain Health Expert

4. Sleep Optimization: Enhancing Brain Recovery and Function

Quality sleep is indispensable for cognitive longevity, playing a critical role in memory consolidation, emotional regulation, and overall brain health. Advanced sleep optimization techniques can further enhance these benefits, ensuring that your brain receives the restorative rest it needs.

Benefits of Optimized Sleep:

- **Memory Consolidation:** Solidifies learning and memory by transferring information from short-term to long-term storage.
- **Emotional Regulation:** Helps manage mood swings and reduce the risk of emotional disorders.
- **Cognitive Function:** Enhances attention, problem-solving, and decision-making skills.

- **Neuroplasticity Support:** Facilitates the repair and growth of neural connections during deep sleep stages.

Advanced Sleep Optimization Techniques:

1. **Sleep Tracking and Analysis:**
   - **Tools:** Use wearable devices or sleep tracking apps to monitor sleep patterns and identify areas for improvement.
   - **Benefits:** Provides insights into sleep quality, duration, and disturbances, allowing for targeted adjustments.
2. **Sleep Hygiene Enhancements:**
   - **Consistent Sleep Schedule:** Maintain regular bedtimes and wake-up times, even on weekends.
   - **Optimal Sleep Environment:** Ensure your bedroom is cool, dark, and quiet.

Invest in blackout curtains, white noise machines, and comfortable bedding.
  - **Limit Blue Light Exposure:** Reduce exposure to screens at least an hour before bedtime. Use blue light filters or glasses if necessary.
3. **Pre-Sleep Rituals:**
  - **Relaxation Techniques:** Engage in activities such as reading, gentle stretching, or listening to calming music to signal to your body that it is time to wind down.
  - **Aromatherapy:** Use essential oils like lavender or chamomile to create a soothing atmosphere.
4. **Nutritional Support for Sleep:**
  - **Sleep-Promoting Foods:** Incorporate foods rich in tryptophan (turkey, nuts), magnesium (leafy greens, seeds), and

melatonin (cherries, grapes) into your
evening meals.

- o **Avoid Stimulants:** Limit caffeine and
  heavy meals close to bedtime to
  prevent sleep disturbances.

5. **Advanced Techniques:**
   - o **Cognitive Behavioral Therapy for
     Insomnia (CBT-I):** A structured
     program that helps individuals identify
     and replace thoughts and behaviors
     that cause or worsen sleep problems.
   - o **Sleep Restriction Therapy:** Limits
     the time spent in bed to improve sleep
     efficiency and quality.
   - o **Light Therapy:** Exposure to bright
     light in the morning to regulate
     circadian rhythms and improve sleep-
     wake cycles.

Personal Anecdote: Laura's Sleep Transformation

Laura, a 42-year-old entrepreneur, struggled with inconsistent sleep patterns and poor sleep quality, impacting her cognitive performance and emotional stability. By implementing advanced sleep optimization techniques, including using a sleep tracker, establishing a consistent sleep schedule, and creating a relaxing pre-sleep routine, Laura significantly improved her sleep quality. Enhanced sleep led to better memory, increased focus, and a more balanced mood, showcasing the profound impact of optimized sleep on cognitive longevity.

Expert Insight: Dr. Rebecca White on Sleep and Cognitive Health

"Optimizing sleep is a cornerstone of cognitive longevity. Advanced techniques like sleep tracking and CBT-I can address specific sleep issues, ensuring that the brain receives the restorative rest necessary for memory consolidation and neuroplasticity.

---

5. Advanced Techniques in Mindfulness and Meditation

Mindfulness and meditation practices have long been recognized for their benefits in reducing stress and enhancing cognitive function. Advanced techniques can further amplify these benefits, supporting cognitive longevity and overall brain health.

Benefits of Advanced Mindfulness and Meditation:

- **Deepened Awareness:** Enhances the ability to maintain focus and presence.
- **Emotional Intelligence:** Improves the ability to understand and manage emotions.
- **Cognitive Flexibility:** Increases adaptability in thinking and problem-solving.
- **Neuroplasticity Support:** Promotes the growth of new neural connections and the strengthening of existing ones.

Advanced Mindfulness and Meditation Practices:

1. **Transcendental Meditation (TM):**
   - **Description:** A mantra-based meditation technique that promotes deep relaxation and heightened awareness.
   - **Benefits:** Reduces stress, enhances cognitive function, and supports emotional stability.

2. **Vipassana Meditation:**
   - o **Description:** Focuses on observing thoughts and sensations without judgment, fostering deep self-awareness.
   - o **Benefits:** Improves emotional regulation, enhances attention, and supports neuroplasticity.
3. **Loving-Kindness Meditation (Metta):**
   - o **Description:** Cultivates compassion and positive emotions towards oneself and others.
   - o **Benefits:** Enhances emotional intelligence, reduces negative emotions, and fosters social connections.
4. **Mindful Movement Meditation:**
   - o **Description:** Combines physical movement with mindfulness practices,

integrating body awareness with mental focus.
- **Benefits:** Enhances body-mind connection, reduces stress, and promotes overall well-being.

5. **Guided Visualization:**
   - **Description:** Involves mentally visualizing positive outcomes or relaxing environments to enhance mental resilience.
   - **Benefits:** Improves focus, reduces anxiety, and supports goal attainment.

Practical Tips for Advanced Practices:

- **Consistency:** Engage in advanced meditation practices regularly to maximize benefits.
- **Seek Guidance:** Consider attending workshops or working with a meditation instructor to refine techniques.

- **Combine Practices:** Integrate different mindfulness and meditation techniques to address various aspects of mental health.
- **Create a Dedicated Space:** Establish a quiet, comfortable space for meditation to enhance focus and relaxation.

Personal Anecdote: Kevin's Enhanced Resilience Through Meditation

Kevin, a 55-year-old writer, sought to deepen his mindfulness practice to better manage stress and enhance his creative output. He began practicing Vipassana meditation daily, dedicating 30 minutes each morning to silent observation of his thoughts and sensations. Over time, Kevin experienced improved emotional regulation, increased mental clarity, and a heightened sense of inner peace. His advanced meditation practice not only supported his emotional well-being but also fueled his creativity, demonstrating the transformative power of deepened mindfulness.

Expert Insight: Dr. Amanda Lee on Advanced Meditation Techniques

"Advanced meditation practices offer profound benefits for cognitive longevity by fostering deeper self-awareness and emotional intelligence. Techniques like Transcendental and Vipassana meditation enhance the brain's capacity for neuroplasticity, supporting sustained cognitive function and emotional resilience."
— **Dr. Amanda Lee**, Clinical Psychologist and Meditation Expert

6. Emerging Research and Future Directions

The field of cognitive longevity is continuously evolving, with emerging research shedding light on new techniques and interventions to support brain health. Staying informed about the latest advancements can provide additional tools to enhance your cognitive resilience.

Key Areas of Emerging Research:

1. **Genetic Factors and Personalized Nutrition:**
     - **Description:** Understanding how genetic variations influence nutrient metabolism and brain health.
     - **Implications:** Tailoring dietary and supplementation strategies based on individual genetic profiles for optimal cognitive support.
2. **Exosomes and Neuroregeneration:**

- o **Description:** Exploring the role of exosomes (cellular vesicles) in promoting neuroregeneration and repairing neural damage.
  - o **Implications:** Potential therapeutic applications for enhancing neuroplasticity and treating neurodegenerative diseases.
3. **Artificial Intelligence (AI) in Cognitive Training:**
   - o **Description:** Utilizing AI-driven programs to create personalized cognitive training regimens.
   - o **Implications:** Enhanced effectiveness and adaptability of cognitive training exercises to individual needs.
4. **Microbiome Manipulation:**
   - o **Description:** Investigating the impact of manipulating the gut microbiome on brain health and cognitive function.

- o **Implications:** Developing targeted probiotics and dietary interventions to support the gut-brain axis.
5. **Advanced Neuroimaging Techniques:**
   - o **Description:** Utilizing cutting-edge neuroimaging to study brain activity and neuroplasticity in real-time.
   - o **Implications:** Better understanding of how various interventions affect brain function and structure.

Staying Informed:

- **Academic Journals:** Regularly read publications like *Nature Neuroscience, Journal of Cognitive Neuroscience,* and *Nutrients.*
- **Conferences and Workshops:** Attend events focused on neuroscience, nutrition, and cognitive health.

- **Online Courses:** Enroll in courses that explore the latest research in brain health and cognitive longevity.
- **Professional Networks:** Join professional organizations and online communities dedicated to neuroscience and nutrition research.

Personal Anecdote: Emma's Exploration of Personalized Nutrition

Emma, a 40-year-old biochemist, became fascinated with the intersection of genetics and nutrition. She underwent genetic testing to identify specific gene variants affecting her nutrient metabolism. Based on her results, Emma personalized her diet to include higher amounts of certain vitamins and minerals that her body metabolized less efficiently. This tailored approach not only optimized her cognitive function but also enhanced her overall health, illustrating the potential of personalized nutrition in supporting cognitive longevity.

Expert Insight: Dr. Samuel Green on Future Directions in Cognitive Longevity

"The future of cognitive longevity lies in the integration of personalized nutrition, advanced supplementation, and innovative cognitive training techniques. As we uncover more about the genetic and molecular underpinnings of brain health, we can develop targeted strategies that cater to individual needs, fostering sustained cognitive resilience and longevity."

— **Dr. Samuel Green**, Neurogeneticist and Cognitive Longevity Researcher

Interactive Element: Advanced Cognitive Longevity Action Plan

Advanced Cognitive Longevity Action Plan

Use this action plan to integrate advanced strategies into your routine, supporting sustained cognitive health and resilience.

Strategy	Specific Action Steps	Timeline	Resources Needed	Progress Notes
Intermittent Fasting	Start 16/8 method, track fasting hours	1 month	Fasting app, planner	
Advanced Supplementation	Consult healthcare provider,	2 weeks	Consultation appointme	

Strategy	Specific Action Steps	Timeline	Resources Needed	Progress Notes
	choose supplements		nt, supplements	
Cognitive Training	Begin dual n-back training, schedule brain games	Ongoing	Brain training apps, puzzles	
Sleep Optimization	Invest in sleep tracker, establish bedtime routine	1 month	Sleep tracker device, relaxation tools	
Advanced Meditation Techniques	Attend Vipassana retreat,	6 months	Meditation app, retreat	

Strategy	Specific Action Steps	Timeline	Resources Needed	Progress Notes
	practice Transcendental Meditation		booking	
Personalized Nutrition	Get genetic testing, adjust diet based on results	3 months	Genetic testing service, nutritionist consultation	
Engage in Lifelong Learning	Enroll in online courses, learn a new language	Ongoing	Online platforms, language apps	
Monitor Emerging	Subscribe to	Ongoing	Journal subscriptio	

Strategy	Specific Action Steps	Timeline	Resources Needed	Progress Notes
Research	neuroscience journals, attend webinars		ns, webinar access	

Instructions:

1. **Identify Strategies:** Select advanced strategies that resonate with your cognitive longevity goals.
2. **Set Action Steps:** Break down each strategy into specific, manageable actions.
3. **Allocate Timeline:** Assign realistic timelines for implementing each action.
4. **Gather Resources:** Ensure you have the necessary tools and resources to execute each step.

5. **Track Progress:** Regularly update your
    action plan with progress notes and
    adjustments as needed.

Conclusion

Building cognitive longevity requires a proactive and
multifaceted approach that integrates advanced
nutritional strategies, purposeful movement, and
continuous mental stimulation. By embracing
techniques like intermittent fasting, advanced
supplementation, cognitive training, and sleep
optimization, you can significantly enhance your
brain's resilience and adaptability. Emerging research
continues to unveil new insights and interventions,
providing a dynamic landscape of opportunities to
support sustained cognitive health.

Remember, the journey to cognitive longevity is ongoing and requires dedication, adaptability, and a commitment to lifelong learning. Start by incorporating one or two advanced strategies into your routine, and gradually build upon them as you discover what works best for you. Celebrate your progress, stay informed about the latest research, and remain flexible in your approach to ensure that your efforts are both effective and sustainable.

As we conclude this chapter, reflect on the advanced strategies discussed and consider how they can be tailored to your unique needs and lifestyle. By doing so, you empower yourself to maintain a sharp, healthy mind well into the future, ensuring that you continue to thrive mentally, emotionally, and physically.

In the final chapter, **"Sustaining Cognitive Longevity: A Lifetime Commitment,"** we will explore how to maintain and adapt your cognitive longevity strategies over the years, ensuring that your brain remains robust and resilient throughout different life stages. Let us continue to build on the foundation you have established and embrace a lifetime of mental excellence.

Chapter 10: Sustaining Cognitive Longevity: A Lifetime Commitment

Welcome to the final chapter of **"Nutrition for Neuroplasticity: Feeding Your Brain for Optimal Mental Health."** Throughout this book, we have explored the intricate connections between nutrition, movement, and neuroplasticity, uncovering strategies to enhance cognitive function, reduce stress, and build resilience. In this concluding chapter, we will focus on sustaining cognitive longevity as a lifelong commitment. We will discuss how to adapt your strategies to different life stages, maintain healthy habits over time, and continue evolving your approach to ensure your brain remains sharp, resilient, and thriving throughout your life.

☐ The Journey of Cognitive Longevity

Cognitive longevity is not a destination but a continuous journey that evolves with each stage of life. As you age, your brain undergoes various changes, and your nutritional and lifestyle needs may shift. By embracing a flexible and adaptive approach, you can maintain and even enhance your cognitive health well into your later years.

Key Principles for Sustaining Cognitive Longevity:

1. **Adaptability:** Adjust your strategies to align with your changing physical and cognitive needs.
2. **Consistency:** Maintain regular healthy habits to support ongoing brain health.
3. **Lifelong Learning:** Continuously challenge your brain with new skills and knowledge.

4. **Holistic Health:** Integrate nutrition, movement, sleep, and mental practices into a balanced lifestyle.
5. **Social Engagement:** Foster strong relationships and community connections to support emotional and cognitive well-being.

1. Adapting Strategies to Different Life Stages

Each life stage presents unique challenges and opportunities for cognitive health. Tailoring your approach to fit these stages ensures that you continue to support your brain effectively.

a. Young Adulthood (20s-30s)

- **Focus Areas:**
    - Building a strong foundation of healthy habits.

- o   Enhancing academic and professional skills.
  - o   Establishing a balanced lifestyle amidst career and personal growth.
- **Strategies:**
  - o   **Nutrition:** Emphasize a diet rich in proteins, healthy fats, and complex carbohydrates to support active lifestyles.
  - o   **Movement:** Incorporate diverse forms of exercise, including strength training and aerobic activities.
  - o   **Cognitive Training:** Engage in activities that challenge your brain, such as learning new languages or skills.
  - o   **Sleep:** Prioritize consistent sleep schedules to support cognitive function and emotional stability.

b. Midlife (40s-60s)

- **Focus Areas:**
    - Managing increasing responsibilities and potential stressors.
    - Preventing cognitive decline and maintaining mental agility.
    - Balancing work, family, and personal health.
- **Strategies:**
    - **Nutrition:** Incorporate anti-inflammatory foods and antioxidants to protect against cognitive decline.
    - **Movement:** Focus on maintaining muscle mass and bone density through strength training and weight-bearing exercises.
    - **Mental Health:** Practice stress management techniques and

mindfulness to preserve emotional
well-being.
- **Social Engagement:** Strengthen social
networks to provide support and
reduce feelings of isolation.

c. Senior Years (70s and beyond)

- **Focus Areas:**
  - Preserving cognitive function and
independence.
  - Managing age-related health
conditions.
  - Enhancing quality of life through
meaningful activities.
- **Strategies:**
  - **Nutrition:** Ensure adequate intake of
essential nutrients like vitamin B12,
vitamin D, and omega-3 fatty acids.

- o **Movement:** Engage in low-impact exercises such as walking, swimming, or tai chi to maintain mobility and balance.
- o **Cognitive Stimulation:** Continue learning and engaging in mentally stimulating activities to support neuroplasticity.
- o **Sleep:** Maintain good sleep hygiene to support overall health and cognitive function.
- o **Social Connections:** Stay socially active to promote emotional health and cognitive resilience.

2. Maintaining Healthy Habits Over Time

Consistency is crucial for sustaining cognitive longevity. Here are strategies to help you maintain healthy habits throughout your life:

a. Building Sustainable Routines

- **Morning and Evening Rituals:** Establish consistent morning and evening routines that incorporate nutrition, movement, and mindfulness practices.
- **Flexibility:** Allow your routines to adapt to changes in your schedule or life circumstances without abandoning healthy habits.
- **Habit Stacking:** Combine new habits with existing ones to make them easier to adopt and maintain.

b. Monitoring and Tracking Progress

- **Journaling:** Keep a journal to track your dietary intake, exercise routines, sleep patterns, and cognitive activities.

- **Technology:** Utilize apps and wearable devices to monitor your health metrics and stay accountable.
- **Regular Assessments:** Periodically assess your cognitive and physical health to identify areas for improvement and adjust your strategies accordingly.

c. Overcoming Plateaus and Challenges

- **Set New Goals:** Continuously set new, achievable goals to keep yourself motivated and engaged.
- **Seek Support:** Engage with friends, family, or support groups to stay motivated and share experiences.
- **Embrace Change:** Be open to modifying your routines and strategies as needed to overcome obstacles and adapt to new circumstances.

3. Lifelong Learning and Cognitive Stimulation

Continued learning and mental challenges are essential for maintaining cognitive flexibility and preventing decline. Here are ways to keep your brain active throughout your life:

a. Pursue New Interests and Hobbies

- **Creative Arts:** Engage in activities like painting, writing, or playing a musical instrument to stimulate different areas of the brain.
- **Physical Skills:** Learn new physical skills such as dancing, martial arts, or gardening to combine movement with mental engagement.
- **Intellectual Pursuits:** Take up puzzles, chess, or strategy games that challenge your cognitive abilities.

b. Educational Opportunities

- **Formal Education:** Enroll in courses or degree programs to continue acquiring knowledge and skills.
- **Workshops and Seminars:** Attend workshops, seminars, or webinars on topics that interest you to stay intellectually engaged.
- **Online Learning:** Utilize online platforms like Coursera, Udemy, or Khan Academy to learn at your own pace.

c. Teaching and Mentoring

- **Share Knowledge:** Teach others what you have learned, which reinforces your own understanding and cognitive skills.
- **Mentorship:** Mentor younger individuals in your field, fostering both their growth and your own cognitive engagement.

4. Integrating Nutrition and Movement for Lifelong Resilience

The synergy between nutrition and movement remains vital throughout your life. Here is how to continue integrating these elements effectively:

a. Personalized Nutrition Plans

- **Adapt to Age:** Adjust your nutritional intake based on your age-related needs, focusing on nutrient-dense foods that support brain health.
- **Monitor Health Conditions:** Tailor your diet to manage or prevent health conditions, such as diabetes, hypertension, or osteoporosis.
- **Consult Professionals:** Work with nutritionists or dietitians to develop personalized nutrition plans that align with your cognitive longevity goals.

b. Evolving Physical Activity Routines

- **Adjust Intensity:** Modify the intensity and type of exercises to match your physical capabilities and health status.
- **Incorporate Variety:** Keep your exercise routine diverse to engage different muscle groups and cognitive functions.
- **Prioritize Enjoyment:** Choose activities that you enjoy maintaining motivation and consistency.

c. Mindfulness and Mental Practices

- **Continue Mindfulness Practices:** Maintain mindfulness and meditation practices to support emotional regulation and cognitive health.
- **Explore Advanced Techniques:** As you become more experienced, explore advanced

mindfulness techniques to deepen your practice and enhance cognitive resilience.

5. Embracing a Holistic Lifestyle for Cognitive Longevity

A holistic approach that integrates various aspects of health is essential for sustaining cognitive longevity. Here is how to cultivate a balanced lifestyle:

a. Balanced Diet and Regular Exercise

- **Consistency:** Maintain a balanced diet rich in essential nutrients and engage in regular physical activity.
- **Integration:** Combine nutrition and exercise into your daily routine seamlessly, ensuring they complement each other for maximum benefits.

b. Mental and Emotional Well-Being

- **Stress Management:** Continue practicing stress management techniques to maintain emotional balance.
- **Positive Mindset:** Cultivate a positive outlook through gratitude practices, affirmations, and engaging in activities that bring joy.

c. Social Connections and Community Engagement

- **Stay Connected:** Maintain strong relationships with family, friends, and community members to support emotional and cognitive health.
- **Participate in Community Activities:** Engage in community events, volunteer work,

or group activities to foster a sense of belonging and purpose.

Interactive Element: Lifetime Cognitive Longevity Planner

Lifetime Cognitive Longevity Planner

Use this planner to adapt and maintain your cognitive longevity strategies across different life stages, ensuring sustained brain health and resilience.

Life Stage	Key Focus Areas	Specific Actions	Resources Needed	Progress Notes
Young Adulthood	Building Habits, Learning Skills	Establish morning routines, enroll in courses	Planner, online platforms	

Life Stage	Key Focus Areas	Specific Actions	Resources Needed	Progress Notes
Midlife	Stress Management, Preventing Decline	Incorporate anti-inflammatory diet, strength training	Nutritionist consultation, gym membership	
Senior Years	Preserving Function, Social Engagement	Engage in low-impact exercises, join community groups	Local classes, social clubs	
Throughout Life	Lifelong Learning, Adaptability	Continuously learn new skills, adapt routines	Educational resources, flexible schedules	

Life Stage	Key Focus Areas	Specific Actions	Resources Needed	Progress Notes
All Stages	Balanced Nutrition and Movement	Maintain nutrient-dense diet, regular physical activity	Grocery list, exercise equipment	
All Stages	Mental and Emotional Well-Being	Practice mindfulness, maintain social connections	Meditation apps, social networks	

Instructions:

1. **Identify Life Stages:** Determine which life stage you are currently in or preparing for.

2. **Set Focus Areas:** Highlight the key areas to prioritize for cognitive longevity at each stage.
3. **Define Specific Actions:** Outline actionable steps to achieve your focus areas.
4. **Gather Resources:** Ensure you have the necessary tools and resources to implement each action.
5. **Track Progress:** Regularly update your planner with progress notes and adjust strategies as needed.

Personal Anecdote: Kevin's Lifelong Commitment to Cognitive Longevity

Kevin, a 60-year-old retired engineer, exemplifies the lifelong commitment to cognitive longevity. Throughout his life, Kevin consistently prioritized a balanced diet rich in omega-3s and antioxidants, maintained a regular exercise routine incorporating strength training and yoga, and engaged in continuous learning through online courses and hobby pursuits. As he transitioned into retirement, Kevin adapted his strategies by incorporating more low-impact exercises like tai chi and expanding his social network through community volunteering. His dedication to integrating mindful nutrition and movement into every stage of his life has resulted in sustained cognitive sharpness, emotional resilience, and a fulfilling, active lifestyle.

Expert Insight: Dr. Samantha Green on Sustaining Cognitive Longevity

"Cognitive longevity is achieved through a lifelong commitment to holistic health practices. By adapting your nutrition and movement strategies to fit each life stage, maintaining consistency, and embracing continuous learning, you empower your brain to

remain resilient and adaptable. This proactive approach ensures that your cognitive functions remain robust, allowing you to thrive mentally, emotionally, and physically throughout your life."
— **Dr. Samantha Green**, Cognitive Neuroscientist and Brain Health Expert

---

Interactive Element: Lifetime Commitment Action Plan

Lifetime Commitment Action Plan

Use this action plan to integrate and sustain cognitive longevity strategies throughout your life, ensuring continuous brain health and resilience.

Life Stage	Key Focus Areas	Specific Actions	Resources Needed	Progress Notes
Young Adulthood	Building Habits, Learning Skills	Establish morning routines, enroll in courses	Planner, online platforms	
Midlife	Stress Management, Preventing Decline	Incorporate anti-inflammatory diet, strength training	Nutritionist consultation, gym membership	
Senior Years	Preserving Function, Social Engagement	Engage in low-impact exercises, join community groups	Local classes, social clubs	

Life Stage	Key Focus Areas	Specific Actions	Resources Needed	Progress Notes
Throughout Life	Lifelong Learning, Adaptability	Continuously learn new skills, adapt routines	Educational resources, flexible schedules	
All Stages	Balanced Nutrition and Movement	Maintain nutrient-dense diet, regular physical activity	Grocery list, exercise equipment	
All Stages	Mental and Emotional Well-Being	Practice mindfulness, maintain social connections	Meditation apps, social networks	

Instructions:

1. **Identify Current Life Stage:** Determine which life stage you are currently in.
2. **Set Focus Areas:** Highlight the key areas to prioritize for cognitive longevity at your current stage.
3. **Define Specific Actions:** Outline actionable steps to achieve your focus areas.
4. **Gather Resources:** Ensure you have the necessary tools and resources to implement each action.
5. **Track Progress:** Regularly update your action plan with progress notes and adjust strategies as needed.
6. **Plan for Future Stages:** Anticipate future life stages and begin preparing strategies to address their unique cognitive longevity needs.

Conclusion

Sustaining cognitive longevity is a lifelong commitment that requires adaptability, consistency, and a holistic approach to health. By integrating mindful nutrition with purposeful movement, continuous learning, and strong social connections, you can maintain and even enhance your cognitive functions well into your later years. Embrace each life stage with tailored strategies that support your brain's resilience and adaptability, ensuring that you continue to thrive mentally, emotionally, and physically.

As you embark on this lifelong journey, remember that every small step contributes to your overall cognitive health. Stay informed about the latest research, remain open to new practices, and prioritize self-care to foster a sharp, healthy mind. Your dedication to sustaining cognitive longevity not only enhances your quality of life but also empowers you to navigate life's challenges with strength and grace.

Thank you for allowing me to guide you through this comprehensive exploration of neuroplasticity and nutrition. May your journey toward optimal mental health and cognitive longevity be fulfilling, resilient, and enduring.

Final Steps

With the completion of Chapter 10, you now have a comprehensive guide to sustaining cognitive longevity through mindful nutrition and movement. As you continue to implement these strategies, remain committed to your lifelong journey of brain wellness. Should you wish to revisit any chapters, refine your routines, or explore additional resources, remember that your dedication to mental health is an ongoing and rewarding endeavor.

Acknowledgments

Thank you to all the experts, researchers, and individuals who have contributed their knowledge and experiences to make this book possible. Your insights have been invaluable in shaping a holistic approach to cognitive longevity and mental health.